ACSM Fitness Book

Second Edition

American College of Sports Medicine

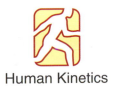

Human Kinetics

Library of Congress Cataloging-in-Publication Data

ACSM fitness book / American College of Sports Medicine. — 2nd ed.
    p.   cm.
    Includes index.
    ISBN 0-88011-783-4
    1. Exercise.   2. Physical fitness--Testing.   I. American College
of Sports Medicine.   II. Title: Fitness book.   III. Title: American
College of Sports Medicine fitness book.
GV481.A322   1998
613.7'1--DC21   97-8611
                                                               CIP

ISBN: 0-88011-783-4

Copyright © 1992, 1998 by American College of Sports Medicine

Acquisitions Editor: Martin Barnard; **Developmental Editor:** Holly Gilly; **Assistant Editors:** Chad Johnson and Rebecca Crist; **Editorial Assistant:** Amy Carnes; **Copyeditor:** Karen Bojda; **Proofreader:** Pam Johnson; **Indexer:** Margie Towery; **Graphic Designer and Graphic Artist:** Stuart Cartwright; **Photo Editor:** Boyd LaFoon; **Cover Designer:** Jack Davis; **Photographer (cover):** The Stock Market/Paul Barton; **Photographer (interior):** Chris Brown; **Illustrators:** Patrick Griffin (cartoons), Timothy J. Shedelbower, and Stuart Cartwright.

Human Kinetics books are available at special discounts for bulk purchase. Special editions or book excerpts can also be created to specification. For details, contact the Special Sales Manager at Human Kinetics.

Printed in Hong Kong by Creative Printing   10 9 8 7 6 5 4 3 2

Human Kinetics
Web site: http://www.humankinetics.com/

United States: Human Kinetics, P.O. Box 5076, Champaign, IL 61825-5076
1-800-747-4457
e-mail: humank@hkusa.com

Canada: Human Kinetics, 475 Devonshire Road, Unit 100, Windsor, ON N8Y 2L5
1-800-465-7301 (in Canada only)
e-mail: humank@hkcanada.com

Europe: Human Kinetics, P.O. Box IW14, Leeds LS16 6TR, United Kingdom
(44) 1132 781708
e-mail: humank@hkeurope.com

Australia: Human Kinetics, 57A Price Avenue, Lower Mitcham, South Australia 5062
(08) 277 1555
e-mail: humank@hkaustralia.com

New Zealand: Human Kinetics, P.O. Box 105-231, Auckland Central
(09) 523 3462
e-mail: humank@hknewz.com

Contents

Foreword

These last few years of the 20th century have been exciting ones for professionals in exercise science and sports medicine. Research, which continues to expand our understanding of the effects of physical activity on health, has recently shown that physical activity and cardiorespiratory fitness are as important to extending longevity as is avoiding the use of tobacco. Studies have demonstrated that improving on low levels of activity and fitness reduces the risk of cardiovascular disease as much as or more than does lowering elevated blood cholesterol or blood pressure. Regular physical activity decreases risk of several chronic diseases, such as heart attack, stroke, diabetes, and some cancers.

In addition to extending longevity and reducing risk of disease, a fit and active way of life helps preserve functioning in older men and women. We are learning that much of the frailty of old age is due to decades of sedentary living habits. Many individuals in their 80s and 90s have been inactive so long that disuse atrophy has led to very little remaining muscle tissue.

The importance of physical activity in preserving health and function has been recognized by major medical, scientific, and public health groups. In 1995 the American College of Sports Medicine (ACSM) and the Centers for Disease Control and Prevention (CDC) released public health recommendations for physical activity. The core recommendation was that "Every U.S. adult should accumulate 30 minutes or more of moderate-intensity physical activity over the course of most, preferably all, days of the week." In the summer of 1996, the U.S. government published two reports including recommendations similar to the ACSM's and CDC's.

The compelling scientific evidence on the importance of regular physical activity to promoting health, preventing disease, and preserving function requires that we give increased attention to helping more Americans become more active more of the time. This will be difficult. Over the past 50 years technology has removed much exertion from our daily lives. Laborsaving devices at home, at work, and at leisure sites have produced a steady decline in daily energy expenditure that amounts to several hundred kilocalories per day. We are unlikely to give up all our modern conveniences, which leaves each of us with two choices. We can remain sedentary and accept an increased risk for disease and dysfunction, or we can find a way to increase daily expenditure.

Increasing energy expenditure can be accomplished with a variety of strategies. The most straightforward of them is to arrange our schedules to include a specific exercise time. The type of exercise does not matter very much. The benefits of enhanced health accrue in proportion to the total dose of exercise. A second approach, which may work better for many, is to re-engineer some physical activity back into daily life. This approach to increasing physical activity has been called lifestyle exercise. The ACSM-CDC recommendation to accumulate 30 minutes of moderate-intensity physical activity each day is a way to obtain a healthful dose of exercise. For example, we can look for opportunities to take short walks, climb stairs, and get up and move about. This may be more acceptable to those who dislike traditional, vigorous sports and exercise or who find themselves too pressed for time.

The second edition of *ACSM Fitness Book* can be useful to you whether you prefer lifestyle or traditional exercise. Full of good advice on the health benefits of regular physical activity, it provides information about specific exercises and activities, helps you increase your motivational readiness, and gives you the behavioral skills to become more active. I encourage you to do yourself a favor and use this material to permanently increase your physical activity and to reap the enormous health benefits that will result.

Steven N. Blair, PED, FACSM
American College of Sports Medicine
(President, 1996–1997)

Preface

The first edition of the *ACSM Fitness Book* provided thousands of adults like you the information needed to begin and maintain a safe, effective exercise program. As in the first edition, this second edition provides a simple, step-by-step approach to developing a healthy exercise habit. It is intended for the adult who is just beginning an exercise program and wants to make sure that the exercise program is appropriate for his or her individual fitness.

Each of the areas of health-related fitness—aerobic fitness, muscular fitness, flexibility, and body composition—is addressed. Individual programs of exercise ensure that you work at an intensity appropriate to help you optimize all areas of your fitness.

To help you meet the goal of improving your health, we've expanded the content to include new motivational techniques to assist you in starting and continuing your exercise program. We've added new information about the benefits of exercise. In accordance with the latest information available from the Centers for Disease Control and Prevention and the American College of Sports Medicine, we've emphasized the health benefits associated with forming a lifelong pattern of participation in moderate physical activity rather than vigorous, high-intensity exercise.

The exercise programs have been clarified, with both new illustrations and new record sheets to make them easier to use. We've changed some of the exercises to reflect the most current information regarding effective exercises for optimizing health. Finally, we've added new information to assist you when you purchase commercially available exercise products.

The information included in this book has been prepared by a team of experts from the American College of Sports Medicine (ACSM). ACSM includes among its more than 12,000 members scientists, physicians, exercise specialists, educators, and fitness professionals dedicated to improving health and physical fitness through appropriate exercise. This book thus provides you with the most current information regarding exercise and your health.

Congratulations on your decision to make regular physical exercise part of your life. We at the ACSM are proud to help you as you move toward a more active, healthier lifestyle.

Susan M. Puhl, PhD
Associate Professor, State University
   of New York College at Cortland
Editor

CHAPTER 1

Life's Better With Exercise

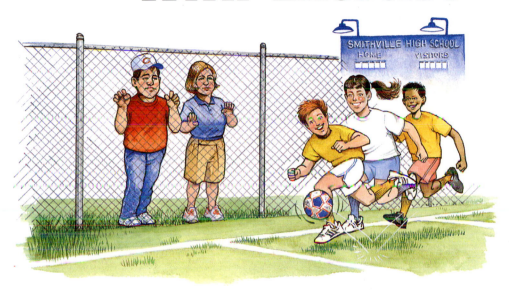

The best reason for beginning an exercise program is that you genuinely want to improve your health and fitness. By reading this book, you're taking an important first step. The decision to make exercise a regular lifestyle habit is a vital one, and an appropriate program can help you do it correctly. Exercise science experts from the American College of Sports Medicine (ACSM) have written this book to help you develop your own healthy exercise program.

The ACSM Fitness Program is designed for the beginning exerciser. The activities are meant for adults who may have been inactive for a few or many years. Even if you consider yourself to be very unfit or if you haven't exercised since you left school, the ACSM Fitness Program can help you improve your health and physical fitness. Best of all, the program takes you *gradually* through a progressive set of exercises. You'll find that exercise need not hurt to be good for you!

If you have already made a commitment to improve your health through exercise and are currently exercising regularly, our fitness assessments will help you determine whether the ACSM Fitness Program is right for you. If the assessments indicate that you're ready for a more vigorous exercise program than the ACSM Fitness Program, the information provided in chapter 5, "The Next Step," will help you select an appropriate and safe exercise program.

The Benefits of Exercise

In the past, exercise scientists and fitness professionals said people should exercise regularly so they'll become aerobically fit. As a result, many people have come to think of exercise programs as being synonymous with vigorous physical activity, like jogging or running. In truth, however, you can achieve many health benefits from more moderate exercise intensities, provided that you exercise often enough and long enough. Moreover, men and women of *any* age can experience these benefits.

Health and fitness benefits increase as the amount of exercise you do increases. But recent research has proved that you can get health benefits from low intensities of exercise— amounts that may not necessarily improve aerobic fitness. The options for such mild to moderate exercise are limitless and include such activities as walking, biking, swimming, hiking, low-impact aerobics, gardening, yard work, and so on.

Exercising for Health

Some of the health benefits associated with regular exercise include lower risk of developing heart disease, adult-onset diabetes, and osteoporosis. And studies suggest that compared with inactive people, those who exercise are better able to cope with stress and are less likely to suffer from depression and anxiety.

Reduced Coronary Risk Factors

Regular exercise can result in modest decreases in body weight and fatness, blood pressure (in people who have mildly elevated blood pressure), blood triglyceride levels, and low-density lipoprotein (LDL) cholesterol, the "bad" cholesterol. In addition, the "good" form of cholesterol, called high-density lipoprotein (HDL) cholesterol, may be increased with as little as 8 to 10 miles of walking per week (or the caloric equivalent of another kind of exercise). However, for optimal improvement in blood fats, regular aerobic exercise should be combined with a diet low in calories, saturated fat, and cholesterol.

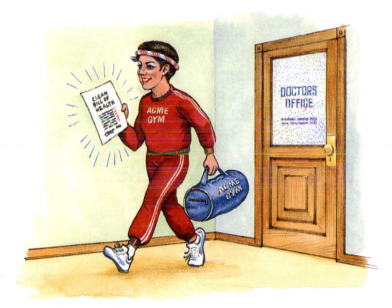

Improved Glucose Tolerance

The ability of the body to regulate the level of sugar in the blood is called *blood sugar tolerance,* or glucose tolerance. When a person's blood sugar tolerance declines, the concentration of sugar in the blood increases, which may lead to diabetes. Approximately one in four older adults is at risk of developing adult-onset, non-insulin-dependent diabetes. Studies have shown that people who are physically active develop this form of diabetes less often than people who are predominantly sedentary. Presumably, regular exercise enhances the body's ability to use insulin (a hormone that regulates the body's use of blood sugar) and to thereby maintain normal blood sugar levels.

Improved Bone Density

Osteoporosis, in which the bones become more fragile over time, commonly occurs in older adults, particularly in women over the age of 50. As a result of the gradual loss of bone mass, even minor falls can cause broken bones, especially at the hip and wrist. It is well documented that weight-bearing exercise such as walking, jogging, and aerobic dance helps maintain bone density. Although improvements in bone density are generally small, it appears that regular exercise, especially muscular strength exercise, also helps prevent further bone loss in persons who are already affected. Such improvements may help prevent bone fractures.

Psychological Well-Being

Many persons who exercise regularly report increased self-confidence, especially in performing physical tasks. Regular exercisers also report these other psychological benefits:

- An enhanced self-image and sense of well-being
- Better sleep
- Less depression, stress, and anxiety
- An improved outlook on life

Many adults find that their opportunities to socialize are limited, and many studies have shown that social isolation is associated with poor general health. Engaging in group activities such as dancing, golf, and water aerobics not only brings people together, but also makes life more fun and interesting.

Exercising for Aerobic Fitness

It's obvious, then, that regular, low-intensity exercise can bring many health benefits. In addition, regular aerobic exercise—exercise that makes your heart and lungs work harder—increases your fitness too. Health-related fitness refers to the ability of your heart, blood vessels, lungs, and muscles to carry out daily tasks and, occasionally, unexpected bodily challenges with a minimum of fatigue and discomfort. Aerobic exercise decreases the heart rate and blood pressure at rest and at any given level of exercise. As a result, the workload (stress) on the heart is reduced.

Research has shown that exercise also increases your ability to take in and use oxygen, which is commonly referred to as the *maximal oxygen consumption* or *aerobic capacity.* Aerobic capacity is a key indicator of your heart-lung function and physical work capacity. When aerobic capacity is high, the heart, lungs, and blood vessels are able to transport and deliver large amounts of oxygen to body tissues. Consequently, your body can produce more energy for occupational or recreational activities, and you won't get fatigued as quickly.

When your aerobic capacity improves, you'll probably experience the following physiological changes:

- The amount of air your lungs can take in increases due to increases in the rate and depth of breathing.
- The amount of oxygen that moves from your lungs to the blood increases.
- Your heart pumps more oxygen-rich blood to the muscles with each beat.
- Your muscles are able to extract more oxygen from the bloodstream.

High aerobic capacity is obviously important to a young athlete who wants to compete in a marathon, but how does it help *you* perform your daily activities? First, recognize that any task requires a certain amount of oxygen. An unfit woman, for example, may use nearly her entire aerobic capacity to accomplish a simple activity like gardening. Although a fit woman will use a similar amount of oxygen for gardening, she will have more energy to tap and be less tired because her aerobic capacity is higher.

Walking is undoubtedly the most accessible and underrated exercise for improving aerobic capacity. Most adults can improve their fitness by regular walking, especially if they are currently inactive.

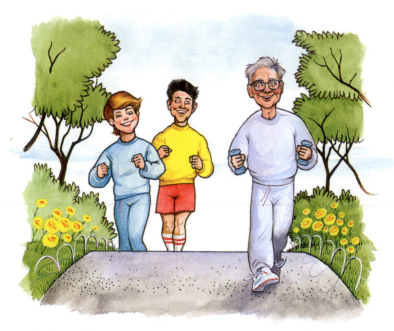

Exercising for Long Life

In the United States, life expectancy in 1900 had not reached 50 years. Today, life expectancy for Americans is approaching 80, and the number of elderly people is growing at twice the rate of the rest of the population. Yet many people often ignore a way of preparing for old age that would help ensure that the "golden years" are long and rewarding: exercise.

Low physical fitness = a shorter life span. That lesson comes from a landmark study that showed that higher levels of aerobic fitness markedly decreased the risk of death from cancer and heart disease. The least-fit men and women in the study had substantially higher death rates than the most fit. But men who progressed from the lowest fitness level to the next category had the biggest decrease in risk! The study emphasized that the fitness level associated with the lowest mortality rate could be easily achieved by most men and women if they would walk briskly for 30 minutes or more every day. These and other recent findings indicate that even small increases in activity and fitness can have a favorable impact on longevity.

Exercise not only contributes to longevity, but it also offers a way to reduce many of the physiological effects that are commonly assumed to be "inevitable" with aging. As people age, they discover that it is harder to do the activities they took for granted when they were younger, so they cut back even more. They accept rides instead of walking a short distance, and they often give up walking for pleasure. This, unfortunately, starts a vicious circle of disuse that makes them even weaker.

There is a close association between chronological aging and physical inactivity. The advancing years typically lead to deterioration in many functions, such as the ones listed in this table.

Effects of Aging and Exercise on the Body and Its Functions		
Variable	**Effect of aging**	**Effect of exercise**
Aerobic fitness	negative	positive
Heart function	negative	positive
Blood pressure	negative	positive
Strength	negative	positive
Resting metabolism	negative	positive
Insulin activity	negative	positive
Blood fats	negative	positive
Bone density	negative	positive
Temperature regulation	negative	positive
Joint mobility	negative	positive
Psychological well-being	negative	positive
Senses*	negative	?
Memory	negative	?
*Hearing, eyesight, taste, smell		

These changes often produce the stereotypical "old" person: the hunched-over, elderly woman who wears sweaters in the summer and can no longer open a jar of pickles or the man whose walk has turned into a shuffle and who is so stiff he can barely bend over to tie his shoelaces. Exercise clearly reduces or prevents many of these adverse changes. The protective and perhaps restorative potential of regular physical activity is a matter of critical importance to billions of people who are moving toward older age.

For example, consider the age-related deterioration in our ability to take in and use oxygen. After the age of 20, aerobic capacity—a key indicator of our capacity to produce energy—typically decreases by about one percent per year. Because an exercise program will usually increase this variable by about 20 percent, the physically active 60-year-old may achieve the same fitness level as the inactive 40-year-old. In other words, regular exercise can lead to a 20-year functional rejuvenation in this respect. The saying "Use it or lose it" seems particularly applicable when it comes to slowing the aging process.

Physical Activity for All

Recently, an expert panel commissioned by the Centers for Disease Control and Prevention and the American College of Sports Medicine reviewed the research on the health benefits of regular physical activity. The recommendations of the panel were expressed in this concise public health message:

> *Every U.S. adult should accumulate 30 minutes or more of moderate-intensity physical activity on most, preferably all, days of the week.*

Whether you're interested in improving overall health, increasing aerobic fitness, or slowing the aging process, it's great advice.

What Is Fitness?

Early in this chapter we said that health-related physical fitness refers to the ability of your heart, blood vessels, lungs, and muscles to carry out daily tasks and occasional, unexpected bodily challenges with a minimum of fatigue and discomfort. In other words, it's having the *reserve* to do all that you want to do—and more!

Fitness means different things to different people. Becoming fit does not require hard physical activity, monotonous workouts, or a health club membership. To be physically fit, you simply need a regular program of exercise.

You need to understand, though, that physical fitness is a lifetime pursuit. A program that lasts 10 or 12 weeks won't bring a lifetime of fitness benefits. Unfortunately, if you stop exercising, your fitness gains will be lost over time.

Health-related physical fitness actually has four components:

 Aerobic fitness—The body's ability to take in and use oxygen to produce energy

 Muscular fitness—The strength and endurance of your muscles

 Flexibility—The ability to bend joints and stretch muscles through a full range of motion

 Body composition—The amount of fat tissue relative to other tissue in your body

Because fitness has different components, the *ACSM Fitness Book* provides you with a physical conditioning program that includes exercises to improve your fitness in all four areas.

Aerobic Fitness

The ACSM Fitness Program uses walking to improve aerobic fitness. Walking offers an easily tolerated exercise intensity and causes fewer musculoskeletal and orthopedic problems of the lower extremities than jogging or running does. It is also an activity that requires no special equipment other than a pair of well-fitted athletic shoes. Other effective exercises that employ large muscle groups can also improve your aerobic fitness. Such activities include stationary or outdoor bicycling, rowing, swimming, skating, stair climbing, and simulated or real cross-country skiing.

Muscular Fitness

Muscular fitness is essential to most of your daily tasks, whether lifting a child or pushing a lawnmower. Manipulating your body and the objects around you requires that you have enough strength to move the things you want to move and enough endurance to hold the items or position successfully. The ACSM Fitness Program uses a variety of exercises to improve both the strength and endurance of the major muscles of your upper and lower body.

Flexibility

All movements require some degree of flexibility. Joints and muscles that are not flexible limit movement and increase the risk of pain and injury. When you improve your flexibility, you help prevent strains and other problems, such as back pain. Regular stretching exercises will help increase your flexibility. The ACSM Fitness Program includes stretching exercises for all the major joints of your body.

Body Composition

Your body composition is based *not* on how much you weigh, but rather on how much of your weight is fat. Excessive body fat can cause musculoskeletal problems and increase your risk of heart disease and high blood pressure. On the other hand, too little fat is associated with other medical conditions. You can have a heavy, athletic physique and have little body fat, or be thin but have poor muscle development and relatively more fat. The ACSM Fitness Program suggests regular walking or other aerobic activities, along with muscular fitness exercises, to favorably modify body composition.

Three Simple Steps to Fitness

The ACSM Fitness Program is designed to help you take the guesswork out of planning a safe, effective exercise routine to enhance all areas of physical fitness. We'll take you through a simple three-step approach to developing and maintaining fitness:

1. Find out where you are.
2. Design a program to achieve your goals—and stick with it.
3. Check your progress.

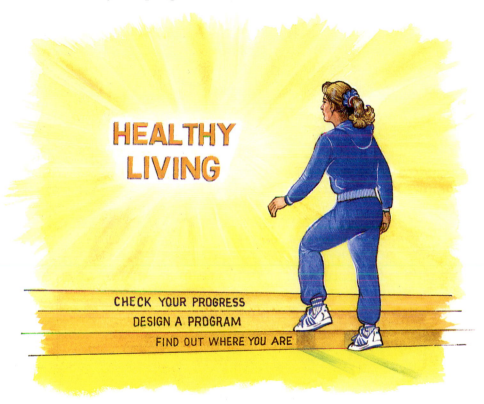

Step 1. Find Out Where You Are

A little later in this chapter, we'll teach you how to set appropriate fitness goals. In order to reach your fitness goals, it is important to know your current fitness status. Otherwise, you might choose an exercise program that is too difficult or too easy for you. In chapter 2, we present a simple four-part test— the ACSM Fitness Test—to help you determine what your fitness is in each of the four components of physical fitness we just described.

Step 2. Design a Program to Achieve Your Goals—and Stick With It!

Your personal ACSM Fitness Program is based on your scores in each of the four fitness components. You'll use the scores to build an individual, color-coded exercise program. You may find, for example, that your test results indicate you're at a higher level in the aerobic fitness component than in the flexibility component. That's OK! The ACSM Fitness Program allows you to choose the exercises that correspond to your fitness level for each component. That way, you can be sure that the exercises are neither too hard nor too easy in any area of fitness development.

Chapter 4 provides easy-to-follow, day-by-day exercise schedules for each fitness level in each of the four components of physical fitness. Each level of the program takes you through six weeks of activity. Each daily schedule includes specific exercises for you to complete. You'll start at the appropriate level for each fitness component and continue until you successfully complete the entire program. When you finish one level of the program, you'll be instructed how to proceed to the next. You'll continue to progress until you've completed all levels of the program or until you've reached your fitness goals. Your fitness will continue to improve in a safe, enjoyable manner.

Step 3. Check Your Progress

Keeping track of your progress in your ACSM Fitness Program is like checking the highway signs on a cross-country trip: It helps you know exactly where you are.

In chapter 4, you'll find record sheets for tracking your exercise progress. Keeping records takes only a few seconds, but it's very important to your total fitness program. It takes the guesswork out of trying to remember what you did and how you felt each time you exercised. Each time you record your progress, you reward yourself! As you work through the program, you'll also want to refer periodically to page 16 to review the goals you've set. When you achieve a goal, reward yourself in some way, then set a new goal. It's easier to stay with your exercise program when you can see the progress you've made.

You Can Do It!

So now you're motivated to begin a fitness program to improve your fitness, be healthier, and live longer. What's the ultimate secret of success? In a word, persistence! Many people exercise for a while, but the results come too slowly, so they quit and go looking for something easier. What they don't realize is that if they had hung on just a little bit longer, they could have reached their goals and reaped the rewards.

Unfortunately, when it comes to lifestyle changes such as exercise, too many people think that it's an all-or-none phenomenon. Nothing could be farther from the truth. Achieving health and fitness is similar to running a marathon, not a sprint. In other words, it's what you do over the long term that really counts. Don't worry about one particular point in the race when you may not have performed as well as you had hoped. All too often, some people give up their exercise program because they failed to follow it perfectly. But people aren't perfect. They mistakenly reason that all is lost, and they go back to their old ways.

By reading this book, you've taken a significant step in making regular exercise part of your life. It's important to realize that the favorable impact on health and fitness that results from a program of exercise occurs only when you stick with the program. While most people can be encouraged to begin a good exercise program, fewer than half the people who start an exercise program actually stay with it. Some people get bored with exercise or don't have the commitment to stick with a program. It might be difficult for them to find a convenient time to exercise, or they become frustrated because they aren't seeing the results of their program as quickly as they want. When it comes to sustaining interest and enthusiasm, these negative variables can really derail a program.

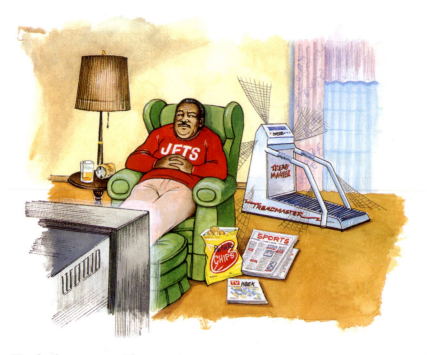

To help yourself maintain your motivation to sustain a regular exercise commitment, first acknowledge this simple yet important fact: Exercise is voluntary and time-consuming. Therefore, it may compete with other valued interests and responsibilities of daily life. Here are several things you can do, beyond relying on mere willpower, to maintain your motivation.

Learn all you can about the whys and hows of exercise.

If you thoroughly understand the benefits that can be derived from following a regular exercise program, you'll be more inclined to stick with it. Good instruction provided by qualified exercise leaders, such as those certified by the American College of Sports Medicine, will give you the knowledge to develop an exercise program that is both safe and effective.

Minimize your chance of injury by choosing mild to moderate exercise.

Too often beginning exercisers become discouraged because their muscles are sore or they've become injured from working out too vigorously or from stepping up the pace too quickly. An excessive exercise frequency (more than five workouts per week), duration (more than 45 minutes per session), or intensity (always working at hard to very hard effort) offers little additional gain in fitness but disproportionately increases the incidence of injury.

A starter program may include just 20 to 30 minutes of exercise every other day at a comfortable intensity (fairly light to somewhat hard). Warm up adequately, and be sure to wear proper shoes and socks.

Establish short-term goals.

Goal setting should be viewed much like climbing a ladder, with emphasis placed on reasonable distances between rungs. Refer back to the section titled "Benefits of Exercise," then set goals that relate to those benefits that are most important to you.

As you set your goals, follow these guidelines:

- *Make your goals challenging, but realistic.* For example, if it presently takes you 18 minutes to walk a mile, an appropriate beginning goal would be to walk a mile in 15 minutes rather than in 11 minutes.

- *Set specific, not general, goals.* Rather than setting a goal "to improve muscular strength," aim to increase the number of push-ups you can do at once from 10 to 15.

- *Set short-term goals.* Set goals that you can reach within a time period that is short enough to keep you motivated. Rather than setting a goal of losing 35 pounds this year, set one to lose 3 pounds this month.

The late Earl Nightingale, a well-known authority on high-level personal performance, claimed that fewer than five percent of all Americans have well-established goals. In the context of physical activity programs, goal setting is a sound and highly effective technique for motivating individuals to exercise. Goal setting can be used to tailor an exercise program to your personal needs. Without it, you won't be able to judge your progress, and you'll be less likely to stick with your program.

Take a few minutes to think about your personal fitness goals. After you've identified some, write them down in the first section of the chart on page 16. As you reach your goals, you can set new ones, recording them in the second section. As you continue in your exercise program, your list will help remind you how much you have achieved.

Date	Personal Fitness Goals
	1.
	2.
	3.
	1.
	2.
	3.

Consider joining a group or exercising with a friend.

Commitments made as part of a group tend to be stronger than those made independently. The stimulus of the group often provides the incentive to continue during periods of flagging interest. Better long-term adherence has been reported in programs that incorporate group dynamics as compared with those in which one exercises alone.

Do activities you enjoy.

When exercise is fun or pleasurable, it will help you maintain motivation.

Complete a fitness assessment periodically to check your progress.

Take a fitness test before you start your exercise program and at regular intervals thereafter to assess your response to the exercise program. Favorable changes in these evaluations can serve as powerful motivators that produce renewed interest and dedication. Chapter 2 explains how to complete the ACSM Fitness Test.

Record your exercise achievements on a progress chart.

Research shows the importance of immediate positive feedback on the reinforcement of health-related behaviors. A progress chart that allows you to record your daily exercise achievements can help with this objective. In chapter 4, you'll find record sheets for tracking your progress.

No time? Consider multiple short bouts of exercise.

Recent studies suggest that multiple short bouts of physical exercise yield similar improvements in fitness as single long bouts do, provided that the total amount of time spent exercising is comparable. For many persons, several short bouts of exercise may fit better into a busy schedule than a single long bout. If you can't find 30 minutes a day to exercise, consider three 10-minute bouts spread throughout the day.

Establish an exercise schedule.

Turn mere behavior into a good habit. Early morning workouts make exercise a priority. You might be tempted to cancel late afternoon or evening workouts because of fatigue or unscheduled meetings or delays.

Try this trick to help motivate you to stick with your exercise program: Buy a large glass jar and display it prominently in your home. Put a coin in the jar for each day you reasonably follow your exercise plan. If you fail to exercise for a scheduled

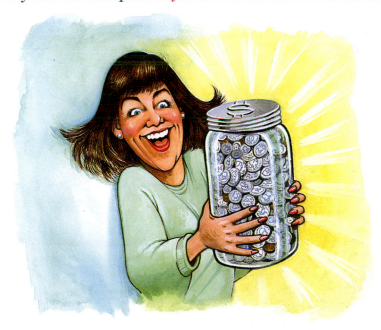

exercise day, take out a coin (or even two), but don't empty out all the precious coins that you've saved to that point. *Then get back on track.* When the jar is full, go out and buy yourself something special. You'll be well on your way to the health and fitness goals that you desire.

We hope you see how easy it will be for you to use this book and to participate in the ACSM Fitness Program. We've done the planning for you, so you can put all your energy into improving your fitness.

CHAPTER 2

Assessing Your Fitness: The ACSM Fitness Test

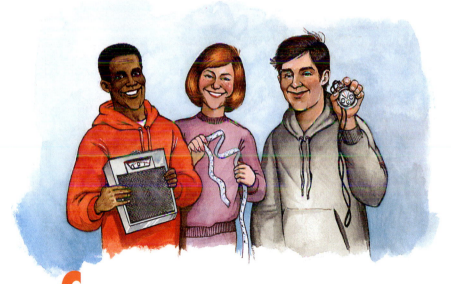

Chapter 1 introduced you to the basic components of health-related physical fitness. Now it's time to discover more about your own personal fitness. This chapter describes the ACSM Fitness Test, a series of four assessments that you can use to evaluate your current physical fitness. The test is easy to perform, and it can be completed in less than an hour. You should enjoy the challenge it offers. As you take the test, you'll record your results for each assessment. Your results will let you know at which level of the ACSM Fitness Program you should begin exercising.

Why Fitness Testing Is a Good Idea

When you begin to exercise, you will anticipate an increase in your fitness. You'll soon begin to feel and function better, but there's much more to it. You found out in chapter 1 that regular exercise produces a variety of important physical changes, but changes are often hard to recognize because they occur gradually. Taking the ACSM Fitness Test at regular intervals will help you identify your rate of progress. It will also allow you to understand the effort required for you to see positive results from your exercise program. As your scores in the ACSM Fitness Test improve, you'll enjoy a great feeling of accomplishment and satisfaction.

Are You Ready to Begin?

The activities in the *ACSM Fitness Book* are designed for adults of all ages who want to begin exercising. For most people, physical activity of moderate intensity isn't dangerous, and no medical clearance is necessary. However, certain individuals should consult with a physician before they begin exercising and before completing the assessments in this chapter. Take a few minutes to answer the questions in the preparticipation checklist on page 21. If you answer "yes" to any of the items, we advise you to seek medical advice about the type of exercise that is safe and appropriate for you *before* you continue with this program.

Gathering Your Supplies

The four assessments that make up the ACSM Fitness Test are the Rockport One-Mile Walking Test for aerobic fitness, a push-up test for muscular strength and endurance, a sit-and-reach test for flexibility, and determination of your body composition through the body mass index and the waist-to-hip ratio. You can complete three of the four items in the ACSM Fitness Test in your own home. The walking test requires a flat,

Preparticipation Checklist

	Yes	No
1. Has a doctor ever said you have heart trouble?	___	___
2. Do you suffer frequently from chest pains?	___	___
3. Do you often feel faint or have spells of severe dizziness?	___	___
4. Has a doctor ever said your blood pressure was too high?	___	___
5. Has a doctor ever told you that you have a bone or joint problem, such as arthritis, that has been or could be aggravated by exercise?	___	___
6. Are you over age 65 and not accustomed to any exercise?	___	___
7. Are you taking any prescription medications, such as those for heart problems or high blood pressure?	___	___
8. Is there a good physical reason not mentioned here that you should not follow an activity program?	___	___

If you answer "yes" to any question, we advise you to consult with your physician before beginning an exercise program.

Note: From the PAR-Q Validation Report (modified version) by the British Columbia Department of Health, D.M. Chisholm, M.I. Collins, W. Davenport, N. Gruber, L.L. Kulak, 1975, *British Columbia Medical Journal*, 17.

measured walking surface, which you should be able to find in one of these locations:

- A neighborhood school or college track
- A community fitness center
- A community park
- A sidewalk along a flat street (You'll have to measure this yourself. Drive your car along the street and note the distance with appropriate landmarks.)

You'll need to gather this basic equipment to complete the assessments:

- A watch with a second hand or a stopwatch
- A tape measure
- A scale to measure your weight
- A yardstick
- Adhesive tape (any type)

It's best to take the test with a friend or relative. You can help each other do the assessments, and your measurements will be more accurate. Taking the tests together is also a great way to involve your friend in your exercise program, and exercising with someone else is an excellent way to ensure that you stick with your program.

To take the ACSM Fitness Test, it's best to wear appropriate clothes and walking shoes, but any flat, comfortable shoes are fine. We recommend a warm-up suit or elastic-waist slacks or shorts and a T-shirt, but any loose-fitting clothing will do.

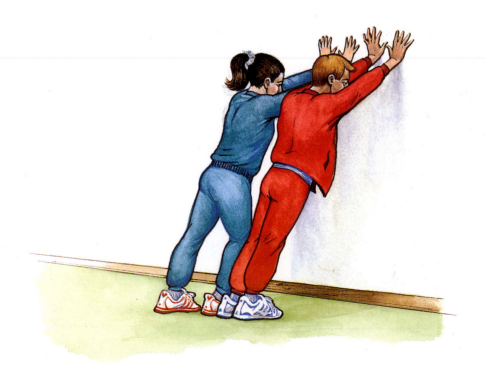

After you have dressed appropriately, gathered all the equipment, and found your measured walking site, you can begin the assessments. As with any exercise, your ACSM Fitness Test begins with an appropriate warm-up. The warm-up is important because it allows your heart rate and respiration to increase gradually, allows your muscles to loosen, and warms your body, all of which should make your assessments and exercise easier. An appropriate warm-up includes these parts:

- Light aerobic activity, such as walking. You can walk in place for a few minutes if you want to perform the warm-up at home.

- Slow stretching exercises, such as those presented in the level 1 flexibility program (see page 112).

Ready, Set, Go!

Have you

✔ written your personal exercise goals on page 16?

✔ completed the preparticipation checklist on page 21?

✔ answered "no" to all of the questions on the preparticipation checklist, or consulted with your doctor?

If so, then you're **READY** to start!
Have you

✔ found a friend or relative to take the test with you?

✔ gathered all of the testing equipment?

✔ warmed up appropriately?

If so, then you're **SET** to begin!

Now, **GO!**
Begin your ACSM Fitness Assessment and Program!

Creating Your Personal Fitness Profile

Just as there are four components of health-related physical fitness, there are four assessments in the ACSM Fitness Test. Assess your fitness in each of the four components. Your fitness may be high in one category but low in another. Determining your fitness in each of the areas will allow you to choose the appropriate exercises for your current status in each area.

As you complete the ACSM Fitness Test, you'll record your results for each component on your personal fitness profile on the next page. Use only the first blank space for each component when you complete the assessment for the first time. As you continue in the program and are ready to retest, record your new results in the other blank spaces. When you're done with the fitness test, the profile will be done, and you'll be ready to develop a fitness program based on your results.

To illustrate exactly how the ACSM Fitness Test works and how you find your results and record your scores, we've invited a pair of new exercisers to go through this process with you. Jackie, 48 years old, and Frank, 37, work together. Recently, a colleague had a heart attack. Realizing it could have happened to them, Jackie and Frank decided to help each other begin and maintain a regular exercise program. They chose the ACSM Fitness Program. Both have followed our instructions so far, and now they're ready to begin the first assessment.

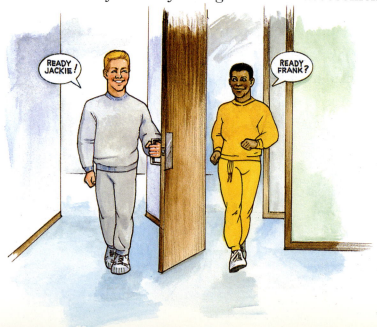

ACSM Personal Fitness Profile
for

_____

Your Name

Fitness Component	Test	Date	Scores	Fitness Level & Color
Aerobic Fitness	Rockport 1-Mile Walk		Time: HR:	
			Time: HR:	
			Time: HR:	
			Time: HR:	
Muscular Fitness	Push-Ups		Number:	
			Number:	
			Number:	
			Number:	
Flexibility	Sit and Reach		Inches:	
			Inches:	
			Inches:	
			Inches:	
Body Composition	Body Mass Index & Waist/Hip Ratio		BMI: W/H:	
			BMI: W/H:	
			BMI: W/H:	
			BMI: W/H:	

Fitness Component 1: Aerobic Fitness
Rockport One-Mile Walking Test

Equipment

- Flat, one-mile walking surface
- Watch or stopwatch

Preparation

- Wear comfortable, loose-fitting clothes and sturdy walking shoes.
- Avoid smoking, eating, and caffeine for two hours before the test. Drinking noncaffeinated beverages is encouraged.
- Practice taking your pulse.

The walking test requires that you count your heart rate accurately. Practice feeling your pulse and counting your heart rate. Your pulse is located at the base of your thumb at your wrist, or at your neck just to the side of your windpipe. Use your index and middle fingers to find your pulse, and count the beats in 15 seconds. Count the first beat you feel as zero. Multiply the number of beats you feel in 15 seconds by 4 to arrive at your heart rate per minute.

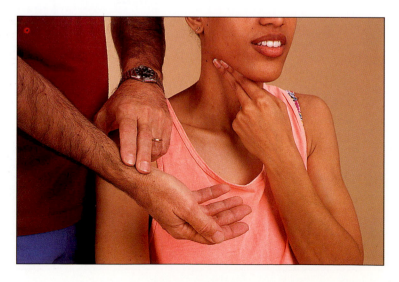

Procedures

1. Warm up by walking slowly for a few minutes then stretching gently using the quadriceps stretch and wall lean shown on pages 80 and 81.

2. Look at your watch to note the time, or start the stop-watch.

3. Begin walking. Complete the mile distance as quickly as you can.

4. Immediately note the time it took to complete the distance.

5. Find your pulse, and count the number of beats in 15 seconds. Remember to count the first beat you feel as zero.

6. Multiply your 15-second heart rate by 4 to arrive at your heart rate per minute.

7. Record your time and heart rate on your personal fitness profile on page 25.

Determining Your Fitness Level

Use the following charts to determine your current cardio-respiratory fitness level.

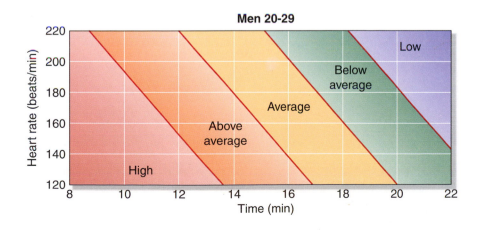

Men 20-29

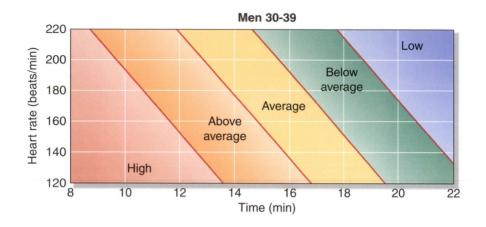

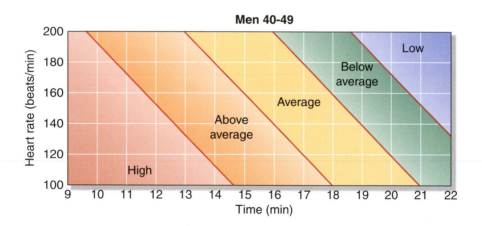

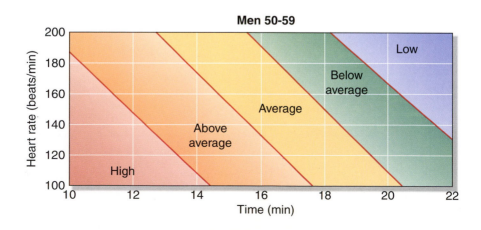

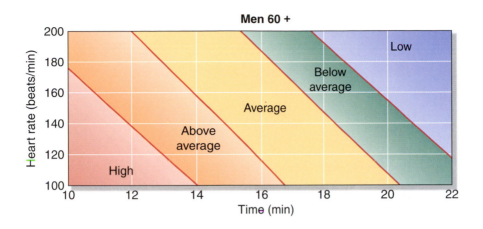

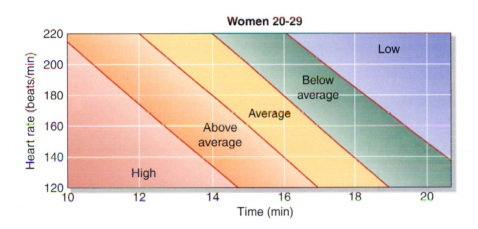

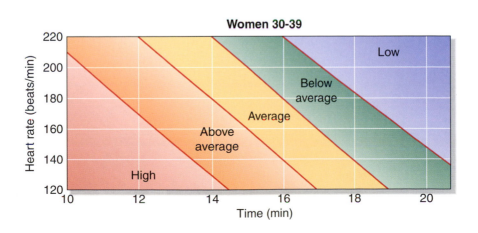

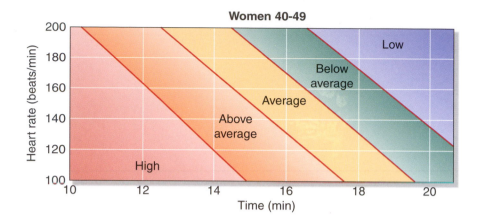

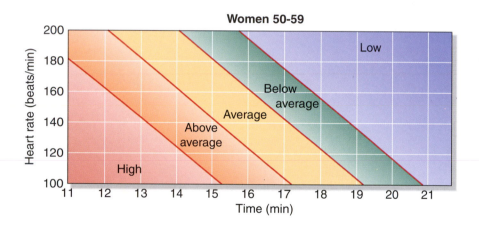

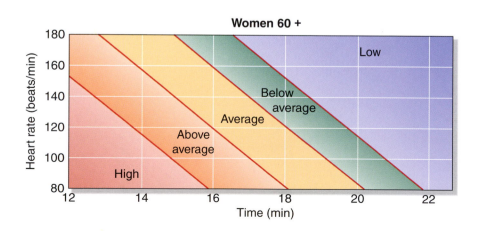

- Select the chart appropriate to your sex and age.
- Find your heart rate along the left side of the chart, and draw a horizontal line across the graph at this heart rate.
- Find the time it took you to complete the distance along the bottom of the chart, and draw a straight line up the graph from that time.
- Read your aerobic fitness level at the intersection of the two lines you've just drawn.
- Once you've determined your aerobic fitness level, record it on your personal fitness profile on page 25.

As Frank warmed up by walking and stretching on the football field encircled by their local high school track, Jackie checked that her stopwatch was working. When Frank finished his warm-up and took his place on the track, Jackie yelled "Start!" and clicked her stopwatch. As Frank began walking quickly, Jackie shouted encouragement. When Frank completed his fourth lap around the track, Jackie stopped the watch and noted that it had taken Frank 17 minutes and 25 seconds to complete the mile walk. As Frank quickly found his pulse, Jackie reset the stopwatch. Again Jackie said "Start," and Frank began to count. At the end of 15 seconds, Jackie asked Frank for his heart rate. Frank had counted 30 beats in 15 seconds. Jackie multiplied the 15-second count by 4 to determine that Frank had a heart rate of 120 beats per minute. Before they left for the track, Frank and Jackie had made copies of the personal fitness profile on page 25. Frank recorded the date, the time it took him to walk the mile, and his heart rate. After Frank had completed his walk and recorded his information, Jackie took her turn walking as Frank operated the stopwatch. Jackie finished walking in 18 minutes and 15 seconds. Her postwalk heart rate was 132 beats per minute.

Frank found the fitness chart on page 28 for 30- to 39-year-old men. Along the bottom of the chart, he found the spot between 16 and 18 minutes. Along the side of the chart, he found where 120 beats would fall. He marked the first spot and drew a line across from the second spot, and he found that they intersected in the yellow area labeled "Average." Jackie found her chart on page 30—the one for 40- to 49-year-old women. Her lines intersected in the green area labeled "Below average." Frank and Jackie recorded their fitness levels and colors on their personal fitness profiles.

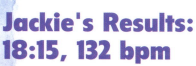

Jackie's Results: 18:15, 132 bpm

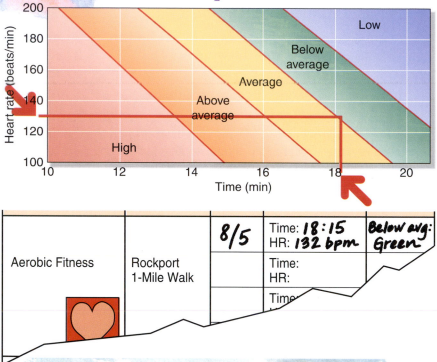

Aerobic Fitness	Rockport 1-Mile Walk	8/5	Time: 18:15 HR: 132 bpm	Below avg: Green
			Time: HR:	
			Time:	

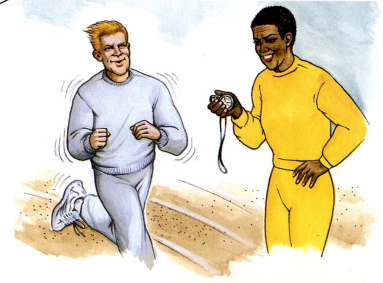

Fitness Component 2: Muscular Fitness
Push-Up Test

Equipment

None

Preparation

- Find a large space on the floor, clear of obstructions.
- Warm up, being sure to use the triceps stretch and shoulder stretch shown on pages 76 and 83.

Procedures

- **Men:** Position yourself on the floor so that your body is straight with your weight supported on your toes and hands. Your arms should be straight with your hands flat on the floor, under your shoulders.
- **Women:** Position yourself on the floor so that your body is straight with your weight supported on your knees and hands. Your arms should be straight with your hands flat on the floor, under your shoulders.

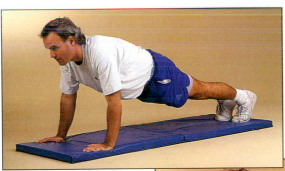

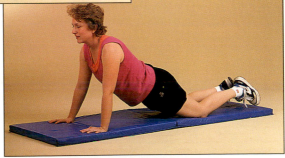

1. Lower your body until your chest touches the floor. Be sure to keep your back straight throughout the push-up.
2. Push your body upward to return to the starting position.
3. Continue lowering and raising your body until you must stop to rest. Count one complete push-up each time you fully lower then raise your body to the start position. Count the number of push-ups you are able to complete without pausing for a rest.
4. Record your score on your fitness profile.

Determining Your Fitness Level

- Compare your score to the standards in the muscular fitness norms table.

Male Norms for the Push-Up Test (number completed)					
Rating	**Age (years)**				
	20–29	**30–39**	**40–49**	**50–59**	**60–69**
Above average	29–35	22–29	17–21	13–20	11–17
Average	22–28	17–21	13–16	10–12	8–10
Below average	17–21	12–16	10–12	7–9	5–7
Low	≤ 16	≤ 11	≤ 9	≤ 6	≤ 4

Female Norms for the Push-Up Test (number completed)					
Rating	**Age (years)**				
	20–29	**30–39**	**40–49**	**50–59**	**60–69**
Above average	21–29	20–26	15–23	11–20	12–16
Average	15–20	13–19	11–14	7–10	5–11
Below average	10–14	8–12	5–10	2–6	1–4
Low	≤ 9	≤ 7	≤ 4	≤ 1	≤ 1

Source: Nieman (1990). Reprinted by permission

Be sure to use the standards for your age and sex.

• Once you've determined your muscular fitness level, record it on your personal fitness profile on page 25.

After the walking test, Jackie and Frank moved to the football field's sidelines to do the push-up test. Jackie went first. She warmed up with the appropriate stretches, then asked Frank to check her position against the one in the photo on page 33. Frank counted as Jackie completed 13 push-ups, which, according to the muscular fitness norms table, indicate she's in the "Average" (yellow) category (she is 48 years old). After Jackie recorded her results on her personal fitness profile, she checked Frank's push-up position and counted for him as he did the test. Frank did 17 push-ups (and he is 37), which puts him in the "Average" (yellow) category, too.

Frank's Results: 17 Push-Ups

Male Norms for the Push-Up Test (number completed)

Rating	Age (years)				
	20–29	30–39	40–49	50–59	60–69
Above average	29–35	22–29	17–21	13–20	11–17
Average	22–28	17–21	13–16	10–12	8–10
Below average	17–21	12–16	10–12	7–9	5–7
Low	≤ 16	≤ 11	≤ 9	≤ 6	≤ 4

Muscular Fitness	Push-Ups	8/5	Number: 17	Average: Yellow
			Number:	
			Num	

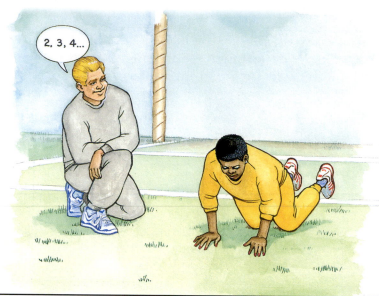

Fitness Component 3: Flexibility
Sit-and-Reach Test

Equipment
- Yardstick
- Adhesive tape

Preparation
- Secure the yardstick to the floor by placing a 12-inch piece of tape across it at the 15-inch mark.
- Warm up, being sure to include the seated toe touch on page 81.

Procedures
1. Position yourself on the floor with the yardstick between your legs (zero mark toward you) and the soles of your feet about 12 inches apart and even with the tape at the 15-inch mark.
2. Ask your friend to position his or her hands across your knees to gently hold them down when you stretch forward.
3. Place one hand on top of the other so that the middle fingers of each hand are even.
4. Gently lean forward along the yardstick, reaching as far as possible. Hold the position for two seconds.
5. Note the distance reached.

6. Relax, then repeat the reach two more times.

7. Record your best score on your personal fitness profile on page 25.

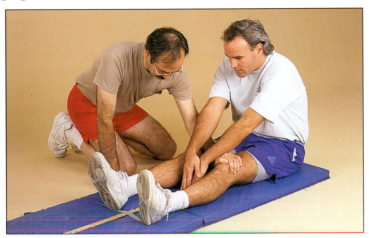

Determining Your Fitness Level

- Compare your best score to the standards in the following sit-and-reach table. Be sure to use the standards for your age and sex.

- Once you've determined your flexibility fitness level, record it on your personal fitness profile on page 25.

Modified Sit-and-Reach					
Score at Age:	20–29	30–39	40–49	50–59	60+
Men					
High	19	18	17	16	15
Average	13–18	12–17	11–16	10–15	9–14
Below average	10–12	9–11	8–10	7–9	6–8
Low	≤ 9	≤ 8	≤ 7	≤ 6	≤ 5
Women					
High	22	21	20	19	18
Average	16–21	15–20	14–19	13–18	12–17
Below average	13–15	12–14	11–13	10–12	9–11
Low	≤ 12	≤ 11	≤ 10	≤ 9	≤ 8

Reprinted by permission, from S. Blair et al., 1988, *ACSM resource manual for guidelines for exercise testing and prescription* (Philadelphia: Lea & Febiger), 165.

Frank and Jackie walked to Jackie's house after they finished their push-up tests. Frank warmed up with the seated toe touch stretch as Jackie taped the yardstick to her kitchen floor. Frank looked at the photo on page 37 and got into the proper position. Jackie held his knees down as he reached forward as far as he could three times, holding for two seconds each time. Frank recorded his best score—six inches—on his fitness profile. He sees in the sit-and-reach table that a score of six for a 37-year-old man puts him in the blue "Low" category. Jackie completed her warm-up while Frank was recording his score, and she was ready to begin. Jackie reached the farthest on the second of her three tries, and she recorded her score of 13— "Below average" (green) for a 48-year-old—on her personal fitness profile.

Jackie's Results: 13 inches

Modified Sit-and-Reach					
Score at Age:	20–29	30–39	40–49	50–59	60+
Men					
High	≥ 19	≥ 18	≥ 17	≥ 16	≥ 15
Average	13–18	12–17	11–16	10–15	9–14
Below average	10–12	9–11	8–10	7–9	6–8
Low	< 9	< 8	< 7	< 6	< 5
Women					
High	≥ 22	≥ 21	≥ 20	≥ 19	≥ 18
Average	16–21	15–20	14–19	13–18	12–17
Below average	13–15	12–14	11–13	10–12	9–11
Low	≤ 12	≤ 11	≤ 10	≤ 9	≤ 8

Flexibility	Sit and Reach	8/5	Inches: 13	Below avg: Green
			Inches:	

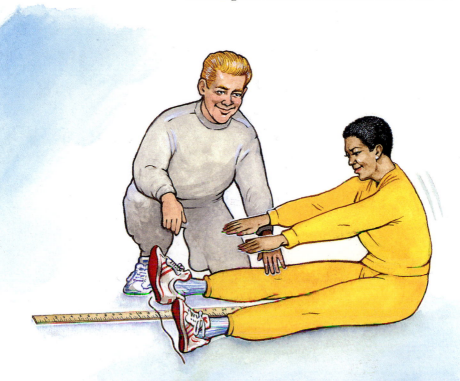

Fitness Component 4: Body Composition
Body Mass Index and Waist-to-Hip Ratio

Appropriate amounts of both fat and lean tissue are necessary for optimal health. However, actually measuring the relative proportion of fat versus lean tissue in your body is extremely complex. We provide two means to help you determine if your body composition is healthy. (But please keep in mind that no single home-based test can provide you with an accurate assessment of your body composition.)

Equipment
- Tape measure
- Scale to measure your weight

Preparation
- Wear minimal clothes and remove your shoes.

Procedures

1. Measure your weight on the scale.

2. Use the measuring tape to measure your height as you stand against a wall with your head, shoulders, buttocks, and heels against the wall.

3. Use the measuring tape to measure the circumference of your hips at the widest part of your buttocks and measure your waist at the smallest circumference of your natural waist, usually just above the navel (belly button). Measure at the end of a normal exhalation without pulling the tape tight.

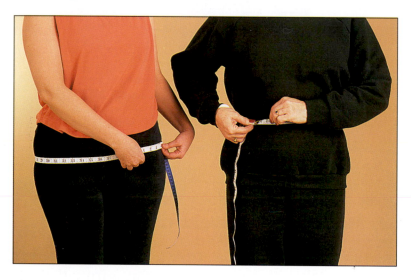

Determining Your Fitness Level

Body Mass Index (BMI)

- Find your weight along the left side of the following chart, and draw a horizontal line across the graph at this weight.

- Find your height along the top of the chart, and draw a straight line down the graph from that height.

- Read your body mass index (BMI) at the intersection of the two lines you've just drawn.

- Record your BMI on your personal fitness profile on page 25.

Body Mass Index Chart

Height (in.)	49	51	53	55	57	59	61	63	65	67	69	71	73	75	77	79	81	83
Weight (lb)																		
66	19	18	16	15	14	13	12	12	11	10	10	9	9	8	8	8	7	7
70	20	19	18	16	15	14	13	13	12	11	10	10	9	9	8	8	8	7
75	22	20	19	17	16	15	14	13	12	12	11	10	10	9	9	9	8	8
79	23	21	20	18	17	16	15	14	13	12	12	11	11	10	9	9	9	8
84	24	22	21	19	18	17	16	15	14	13	12	12	11	11	10	10	9	9
88	26	24	22	20	19	18	17	16	15	14	13	12	12	11	11	10	10	9
92	27	25	23	21	20	19	17	16	15	15	14	13	12	12	11	11	10	10
97	28	26	24	22	21	20	18	17	16	15	14	14	13	12	12	11	10	10
101	29	27	25	23	22	20	19	18	17	16	15	14	13	13	12	12	11	10
106	31	28	26	24	23	21	20	19	18	17	16	15	14	13	13	12	11	11
110	32	30	27	26	24	22	21	20	18	17	16	15	15	14	13	13	11	11
114	33	31	29	27	25	23	22	20	19	18	17	16	15	14	14	13	12	12
119	35	32	30	28	26	24	22	21	20	19	18	17	16	15	14	14	13	12
123	36	33	31	29	27	25	23	22	21	19	18	17	16	16	15	14	13	13
128	37	34	32	30	28	26	24	23	21	20	19	18	17	16	15	15	14	13
132	38	36	33	31	29	27	25	23	22	21	20	19	18	17	16	15	14	14
136	40	37	34	32	29	28	26	24	23	21	20	19	18	17	16	16	15	14
141	41	38	35	33	30	28	27	25	24	22	21	20	19	18	17	16	15	15
145	42	39	36	34	31	29	27	26	24	23	22	20	19	18	17	17	16	15
150	44	40	37	35	32	30	28	27	25	24	22	21	20	19	18	17	16	15
154	45	41	38	36	33	31	29	27	26	24	23	22	20	19	18	18	17	16
158	46	43	40	37	34	32	30	28	26	25	24	22	21	20	19	18	17	16
163	47	44	41	38	35	33	31	29	27	26	24	23	22	20	19	19	18	17
167	49	45	42	39	36	34	32	30	28	26	25	23	22	21	20	19	18	17
172	50	46	43	40	37	35	32	30	29	27	25	24	23	22	21	20	19	18
176	51	47	44	41	38	36	33	31	29	28	26	25	23	22	21	20	19	18
180	52	49	45	42	39	36	34	32	30	28	27	25	24	23	22	21	20	19
185	54	50	46	43	40	37	35	33	31	29	27	26	25	23	22	21	20	19
189	55	51	47	44	41	38	36	34	32	30	28	27	25	24	23	22	20	20
194	56	52	48	45	42	39	37	34	32	30	29	27	26	24	23	22	21	20
198	58	53	49	46	43	40	37	35	33	31	29	28	26	25	24	23	21	20
202	59	54	50	47	44	41	38	36	34	32	30	28	27	25	24	23	22	21
207	60	56	52	48	45	42	39	37	35	33	31	29	27	26	25	24	22	21
211	61	57	53	49	46	43	40	38	35	33	31	30	28	27	25	24	23	22
216	63	58	54	50	47	44	41	38	36	34	32	30	29	27	26	25	23	22
220	64	59	55	51	48	44	42	39	37	35	33	31	29	28	26	25	24	23
224	65	60	56	52	49	45	42	40	37	35	33	31	30	28	27	26	24	23
229	67	62	57	53	49	46	43	41	38	36	34	32	30	29	27	26	25	24
233	68	63	58	54	50	47	44	41	39	37	35	33	31	29	28	27	25	24
238	69	64	59	55	51	48	45	42	40	37	35	33	32	30	28	27	26	24
242	70	65	60	56	52	49	46	43	40	38	36	34	32	30	29	28	26	25
246	72	66	61	57	53	50	47	44	41	39	37	35	33	31	29	28	27	25
251	73	67	63	58	54	51	47	45	42	39	37	35	33	32	30	29	27	26
255	74	69	64	59	55	52	48	45	43	40	38	36	34	32	31	29	28	26
260	76	70	65	60	56	52	49	46	43	41	39	36	34	33	31	30	28	27
264	77	71	66	61	57	53	50	47	44	42	39	37	35	33	32	30	29	27
268	78	72	67	62	58	54	51	48	45	42	40	38	36	34	32	31	29	28
273	79	73	68	63	59	55	52	48	46	43	40	38	36	34	33	31	30	28
277	81	75	69	64	60	56	52	49	46	44	41	39	37	35	33	32	30	29
282	82	76	70	65	61	57	53	50	47	44	42	40	37	35	34	32	30	29
286	83	77	71	66	62	58	54	51	48	45	42	40	38	36	34	33	31	29
290	84	78	72	67	63	59	55	52	48	46	43	41	39	37	35	33	31	30
295	86	79	74	68	64	60	56	52	49	46	44	41	39	37	35	34	32	30
299	87	80	75	69	65	60	57	53	50	47	44	42	40	38	36	34	32	31
304	88	82	76	70	66	61	57	54	51	48	45	43	40	38	36	35	33	31
308	90	83	77	71	67	62	58	55	51	48	46	43	41	39	37	35	33	32
312	91	84	78	72	68	63	59	55	52	49	46	44	41	39	37	36	34	32

Note. Categories are based on values published by the Panel on Energy, Obesity, and Body Weight Standards, 1987, *American Journal of Clinical Nutrition*, **45**, p. 1035.

Waist-to-Hip Ratio (W/H)

- Divide your waist measurement by your hip measurement to determine your W/H ratio.
- From the chart below, determine the risk for adverse health consequences associated with your W/H ratio.
- Record your W/H ratio on the personal fitness profile on page 25.

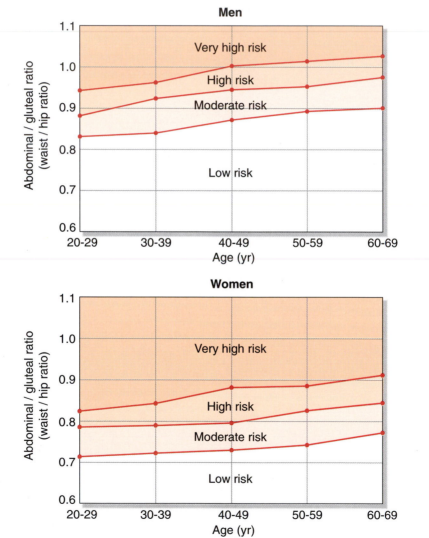

Reprinted by permission of *The Western Journal of Medicine* (G.A. Bray and D.S. Gray, Obesity: Part I — Pathogenesis, 1988, volume 149, pages 429 – 441).

Body Composition Fitness Level

Use the following table to determine your body composition fitness level. Record it on your personal fitness profile on page 25.

BMI category	W/H category	Fitness level
Greater than 30	Very high risk	Green
	High risk	Green
	Moderate risk	Green
	Low risk	Green
26-30	Very high risk	Green
	High risk	Green
	Moderate risk	Yellow
	Low risk	Yellow
19-25	Very high risk	Yellow
	High risk	Yellow
	Moderate risk	Red
	Low risk	Red
Less than 19	Very high risk	Blue
	High risk	Blue
	Moderate risk	Blue
	Low risk	Blue

Note. The fitness categories for body composition are merely indications of the health-risk status associated with your measurements. They are not direct measures of your body composition. As presented at the end of chapter 4 (page 120), you'll use your body composition fitness category to help you determine how often you should exercise.

Jackie brought her scales from her bathroom to the kitchen so she and Frank could do the body composition tests. Both removed their shoes and measured each other as each stood against the kitchen wall. They moved to the scales and weighed each other. Frank, 37, recorded his height and weight. He was 5 feet, 11 inches (71 inches) tall and weighed 178 pounds. Jackie, 48, recorded her results: 5 feet, 6 inches (66 inches) and 157 pounds. According to the body mass index chart, Frank's height of 71 inches intersects with his 178-pound weight at the number 25. Jackie's height and weight of 66 inches and 157 pounds give her a BMI score between 24 and 26.

Jackie's Results:
66 inches, 157 pounds

Height (in.)	49	51	53	55	57	59	61	63	65	67	69	71	73	75	77	79	81	83
Weight (lb)																		
66	19	18	16	15	14	13	12	12	11	10	10	9	9	8	8	8	7	7
70	20	19	18	16	15	14	13	13	12	11	10	10	9	9	8	8	8	7
75	22	20	19	17	16	15	14	13	12	12	11	10	10	9	9	9	8	8
79	23	21	20	18	17	16	15	14	13	12	12	11	11	10	9	9	9	8
84	24	22	21	19	18	17	16	15	14	13	12	12	11	11	10	10	9	9
88	26	24	22	20	19	18	17	16	15	14	13	12	12	11	11	10	10	9
92	27	25	23	21	20	19	17	16	15	15	14	13	12	12	11	11	10	10
97	28	26	24	22	21	20	18	17	16	15	14	14	13	12	12	11	10	10
101	29	27	25	23	22	20	19	18	17	16	15	14	13	13	12	12	11	10
106	31	28	26	24	23	21	20	19	18	17	16	15	14	13	13	12	11	11
110	32	30	27	26	24	22	21	20	18	17	16	15	15	14	13	13	11	11
114	33	31	29	27	25	23	22	20	19	18	17	16	15	14	14	13	12	12
119	35	32	30	28	26	24	22	21	20	19	18	17	16	15	14	14	13	12
123	36	33	31	29	27	25	23	22	21	19	18	17	16	16	15	14	13	13
128	37	34	32	30	28	26	24	23	21	20	19	18	17	16	15	15	14	13
132	38	36	33	31	29	27	25	23	22	21	20	19	18	17	16	15	14	14
136	40	37	34	32	29	28	26	24	23	21	20	19	18	17	16	16	15	14
141	41	38	35	33	30	28	27	25	24	22	21	20	19	18	17	16	15	15
145	42	39	36	34	31	29	27	26	24	23	22	20	19	18	17	17	16	15
150	44	40	37	35	32	30	28	27	25	24	22	21	20	19	18	17	16	15
154	45	41	38	36	33	31	29	27	26	24	23	22	20	19	18	18	17	16
158	46	43	40	37	34	32	30	28	26	25	24	22	21	20	19	18	17	1
163	47	44	41	38	35	33	31	29	27	26	24	23	22	20	19	19	18	
167	49	45	42	39	36	34	32	30	28	26	25	23	22	21	20	19	1	
172	50	46	43	40	37	35	32	30	29	27	25	24	23	22	21	20		
176	51	47	44	41	38	36	33	31	29	28	26	25	22					
180	52	49	45	42	39	36	34	32	30	28	27							
185	54	50	46	43	40	37	35		31	29								
189	55	51	47	44	41													
194		52																

Next, Jackie and Frank measured each other's hips and waists, using the photos on page 40 as a guide for positioning the tape measure. Frank's hips measured 40 inches and his waist was 38 inches. Using a calculator to divide 38 by 40, Frank found his waist-to-hip ratio was 0.95, and his age is 37, which puts him in the "High risk" category. Jackie's waist was 33 inches, and her hips were 42 inches; she is 48 years old. Jackie's waist-hip ratio of 0.79 puts her in the "Moderate risk" category.

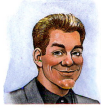

Frank's Results:
Waist: 38 inches
Hips: 40 inches

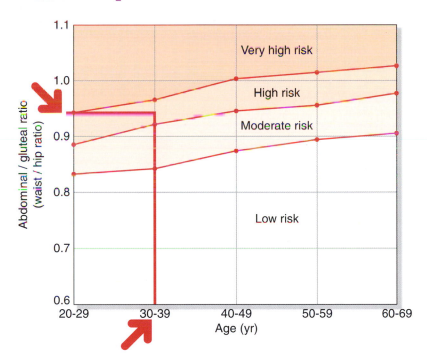

Jackie and Frank used the body composition fitness level chart to find their body composition fitness levels. Jackie, with a BMI score of approximately 25 and a waist-to-hip ratio that's in the "Moderate risk" category, is at the red level. Frank, with a BMI score of 25 and a waist-to-hip ratio in the "High risk" category, is at the yellow level. Jackie and Frank recorded their results on the personal fitness profile.

Jackie's Results:
Moderate risk fitness level

BMI category	W/H category	Fitness level
26-30	Very high risk	Green
	High risk	Green
	Moderate risk	Yellow
	Low risk	Yellow
19-25	Very high risk	Yellow
	High risk	Yellow
	Moderate risk	Red
	Low risk	Red

Body Composition	Body Mass Index & Waist/Hip Ratio	8/5	BMI: 25 W/H: .79	Moderate Risk: Red
			BMI: W/H:	
			BMI:	

With this last entry, their personal fitness profiles are finished.

ACSM Personal Fitness Profile
for

Jackie
Your Name

Fitness Component	Test	Date	Scores	Fitness Level & Color
Aerobic Fitness	Rockport 1-Mile Walk	8/5	Time: 18:15 HR: 132 bpm	Below avg: Green
			Time: HR:	
			Time: HR:	
			Time: HR:	
Muscular Fitness	Push-Ups	8/5	Number: 13	Average: Yellow
			Number:	
			Number:	
			Number:	
Flexibility	Sit and Reach	8/5	Inches: 13	Below avg: Green
			Inches:	
			Inches:	
			Inches:	
Body Composition	Body Mass Index & Waist/Hip Ratio	8/5	BMI: 25 W/H: .79	Moderate Risk: Red
			BMI: W/H:	
			BMI: W/H:	
			BMI: W/H:	

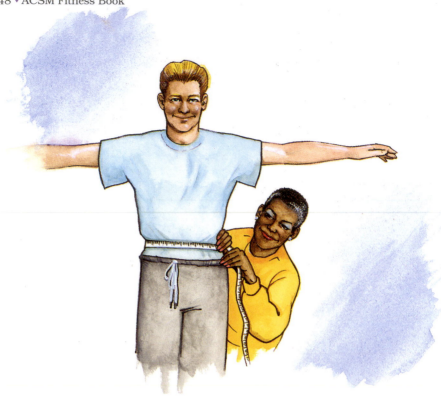

Using Your ACSM Fitness Test Results

Now that you've completed your ACSM Fitness Test, you're ready to begin the exercises designed especially for your level of fitness for each of the components of fitness. Chapter 3 shows you the exercises you'll use in your own personal fitness program. Chapter 4 provides you with daily activity charts to let you know which exercises to perform to ensure safe, gradual improvement in *your* personal fitness.

CHAPTER 3

Beginning Exercises

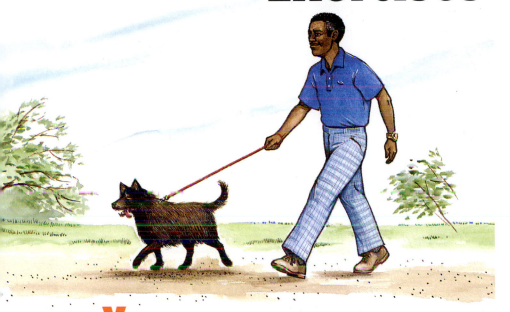

Your commitment to improving your fitness by increasing daily physical activity can begin slowly, simply by being more aware of the opportunities for activity in your daily life. You can walk your dog, play ball with your grandchildren, or mow the lawn.

When you're ready to begin a structured exercise program, you need to determine the specific exercises to include. You may not know which exercises to do to reach your goals. This chapter presents safe, effective exercises that will become part of your individualized fitness program. Exercises for all of the components of fitness—cardiorespiratory endurance, muscular strength and endurance, flexibility, and body composition—are included. In this chapter, we show you the exercises and provide hints on how to derive the greatest benefit from the exercise program. In chapter 4, we help you put the exercises together in programs designed for your personal fitness level.

The exercises in this chapter allow you to gradually increase your fitness. Exercise does not have to hurt to be effective. The old saying "No pain, no gain" is *not* true. Research has demonstrated that you don't have to exercise at high intensity to get positive health benefits.

Here are some general guidelines to follow when exercising for health and fitness:

- Wear loose, comfortable clothing and sturdy shoes.
- Warm up and cool down after each exercise session.
- Exercise hard enough that you feel invigorated but not exhausted. A good way to tell whether your exercise intensity is appropriate is that your breathing rate increases, but you are still able to carry on a conversation.
- Take special care when exercising in hot weather.
  — Slow down your walk or other activity.
  — Exercise early in the morning or later in the evening or in air conditioning.
  — Drink plenty of water before, during, and after exercise.
  — Cool down for a longer period.
- Because exercise is only a benefit if you are feeling well, don't try to exercise when you have a cold, flu, or other illness. Wait until you are feeling better to resume your program.
- If you miss your exercise sessions for more than two weeks in a row, make sure to start out again slowly. Resume your program by repeating the exercises you did a few days before your last workout, then progress normally from that new point.

Exercising for Aerobic Fitness

Many activities can improve aerobic fitness, including walking, biking, dancing, skating, rowing, and other activities that keep your whole body moving in a continuous, rhythmic manner. The ACSM Fitness Program uses walking as the aerobic fitness activity. Walking is one of the best activities. It can be done almost anywhere and requires no special equipment. Walking puts very little strain on the joints and involves all the major muscle groups. It can be done alone or with a group at whatever pace is most comfortable. For all these reasons, walking is one of the most popular forms of exercise. In chapter 4, we give specific daily walking goals as part of your fitness program.

If for some reason you can't or don't want to use walking in your individualized fitness program, you can substitute cycling on an exercise bike or any other aerobic activity. Simply follow the same time guidelines that we've given for walking.

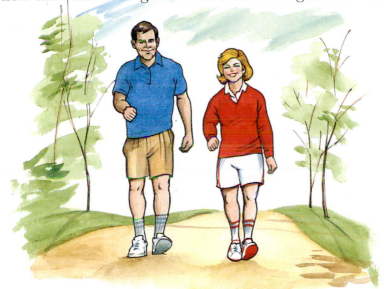

Exercising for Muscular Fitness

A high level of muscle strength and endurance allows you to work longer before you get tired. A combination of exercises is the best way to ensure that you work all of the major muscle groups. We've arranged these exercises by muscle groups. Your own personal fitness program will include some, but not all, of the exercises. The programs in chapter 4 use these exercises; the text in parentheses next to each exercise name tells you what program level the exercise is used in. At the end of the muscular fitness exercise section, we've included some additional exercises that you can use if you want to add a little variety to your muscular strength program.

Many of the muscular fitness exercises can be done with hand or leg weights. Your fitness program is designed to allow you to use additional weight as you progress in your program. Plastic milk, water, or detergent jugs partially filled with sand or water make good weights. The amount of sand or water can be adjusted as your fitness progresses. When using weights, be sure to make all movements slowly. If you experience pain in any of your joints when using weights, reduce the amount of weight, or stop using them.

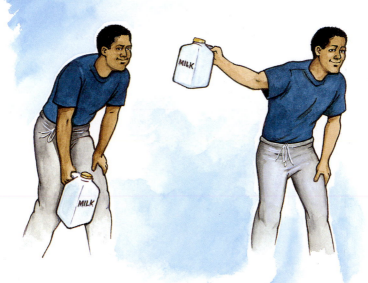

In the past, many women thought they should avoid exercising with weights because they didn't want to develop large, bulky muscles. For most women, this can't happen. Most women's genetic makeup prevents them from developing the large muscles that many men develop when using weights.

Remember these training principles as you complete your muscular strength and endurance exercises:

• Complete all movements in a slow, controlled fashion.
• Maintain normal breathing throughout the exercise.
• Stop any exercise that causes pain.
• Stretch each muscle group after your workout.

ARMS AND SHOULDERS

Wall Push-Up (Level 1)

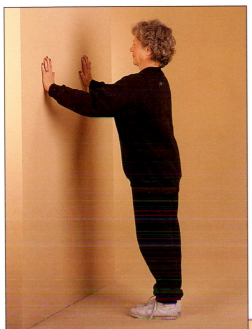

Push body away
from the wall . . .

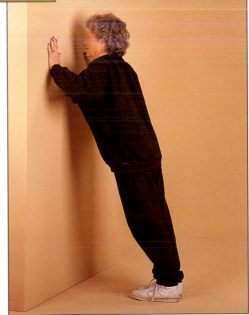

. . . then slowly
lower body to wall.

Chair Push-Up (Level 2)

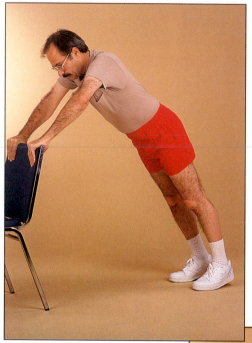

Position the chair against a wall so it won't slide and fully extend arms.

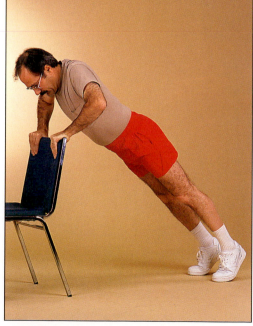

Lower body toward chair.

Knee Push-Up (Level 3)

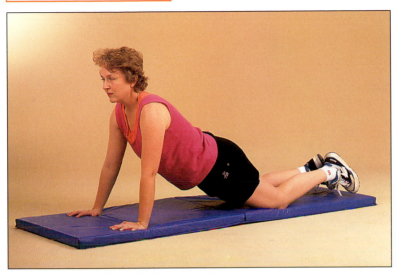

Keep back straight, fully extend arms,
then lower body toward floor.

Toe Push-Up (Level 4)

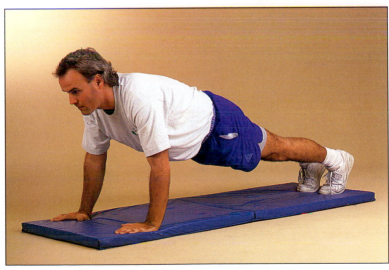

Keep back straight, fully extend arms,
then lower body toward floor.

Single-Arm Row (Levels 1, 2, 3)

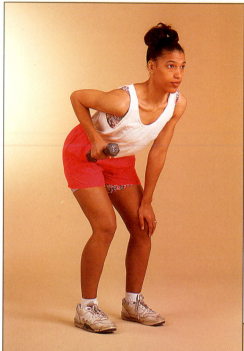

Pull weight to shoulder . . .

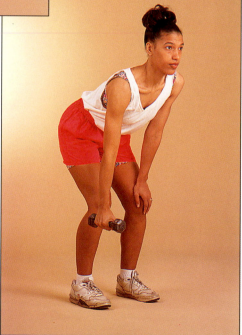

. . . then ease toward floor.

Biceps Curl (Level 4)

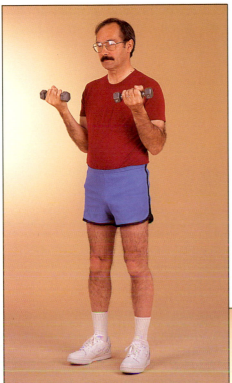

Bending at the elbow, lift weight toward shoulder . . .

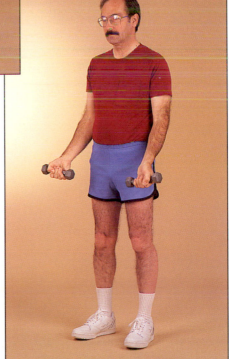

. . . then lower to side.

Reverse Fly (Level 4)

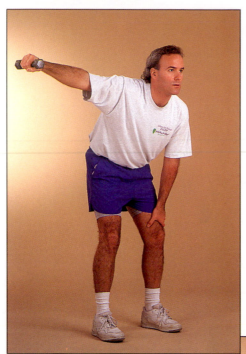

Use shoulder and upper-back muscles to lift weight up and out.

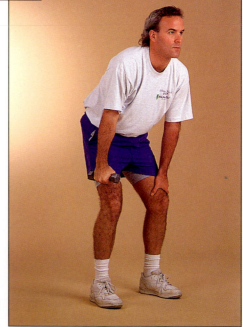

Slowly lower weight toward floor.

LEGS AND HIPS

Seated Lower-Leg Lift (Level 1)

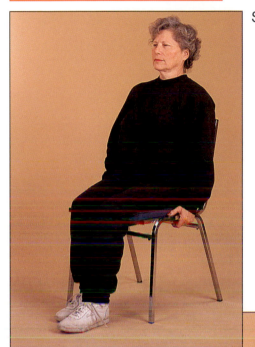

Sit comfortably in a chair.

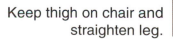

Keep thigh on chair and straighten leg.

Seated Straight-Leg Lift (Level 2)

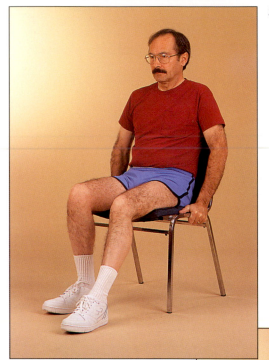

Sit comfortably.

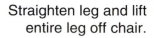

Straighten leg and lift entire leg off chair.

Stair Stepping (Level 3)

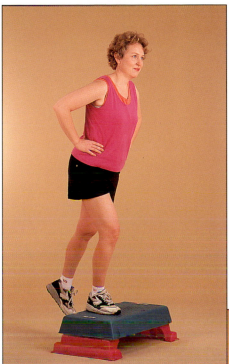

Step up to straight-leg position.

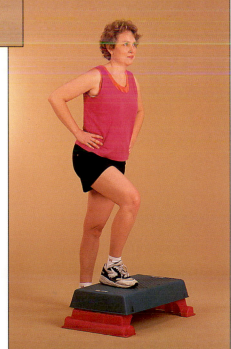

Bend knee to step down.

Chair Squat (Level 4)

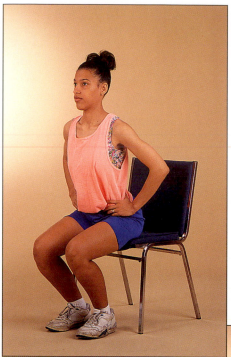

Sit at edge of chair and place heels under seat.

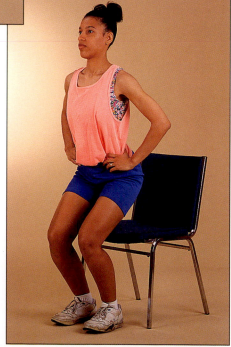

Stand without leaning forward.

Toe Raise (Levels 2, 4)

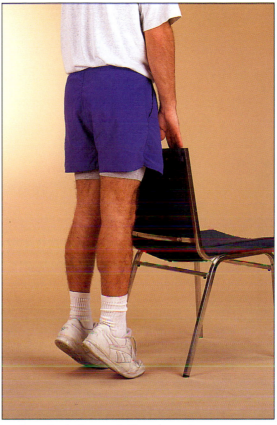

Use the back of a chair for stability; stand on toes, then lower heels to the floor.

ABDOMINALS

Neck Curl-Up (Level 1)

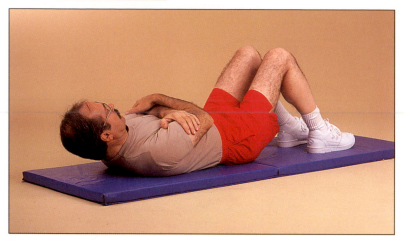

Keep arms crossed; lift head off floor.

Shoulder Curl-Up (Level 2)

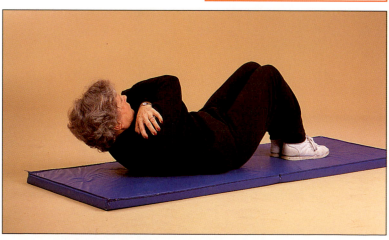

Keep arms crossed; lift top of shoulders off floor.

Straight-Arm Curl-Up (Level 3)

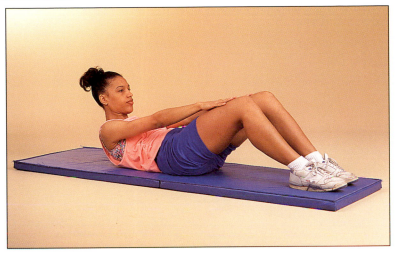

Place hands on thighs; lift shoulders off floor.

Crossed-Arm Curl-Up (Level 4)

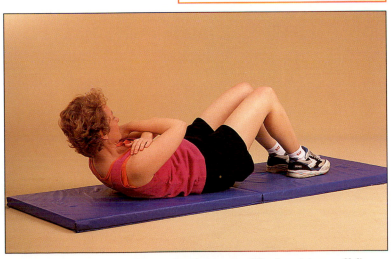

Cross arms; keep chin tucked as you lift shoulders off floor.

BACK

Prone Neck Lift (Level 2)

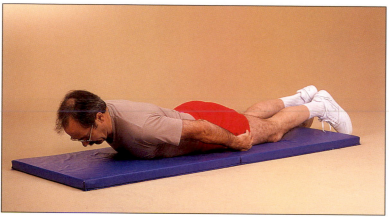

Keep your neck straight as you lift your forehead off the floor.

Prone Single-Leg Lift (Level 3)

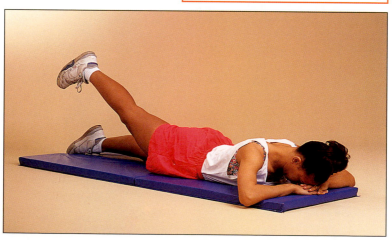

Lift the entire leg from the hip.

Prone Head and Leg Lift (Level 4)

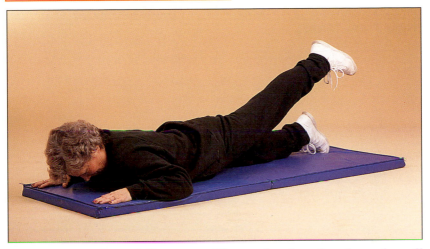

Keep your neck straight as you lift your forehead and one leg off the floor.

ADDITIONAL RECOMMENDED EXERCISES

Triceps Press (Arms)

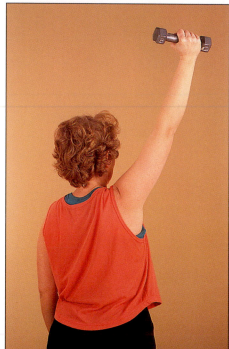

Keep elbow high.

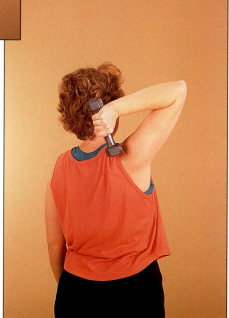

Lift and lower weight
behind your head.

Lateral Raise (Shoulders)

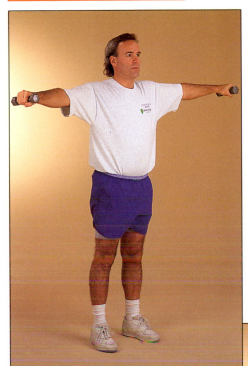

Keep elbows slightly bent as you lift . . .

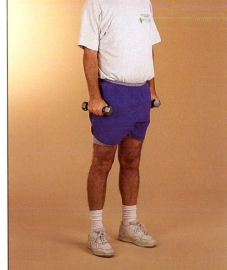

. . . and lower weights
to the side.

Shrug (Shoulders and Upper Back)

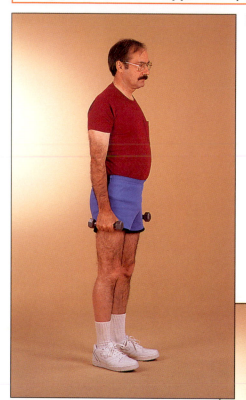

Keep arms straight.

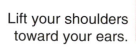

Lift your shoulders
toward your ears.

Inner-Leg Lift (Legs)

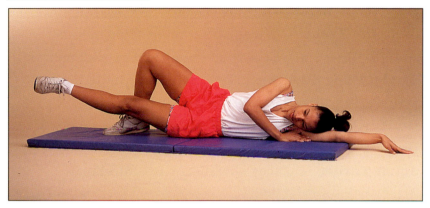

Lift lower leg off floor.

Outer-Leg Lift (Legs)

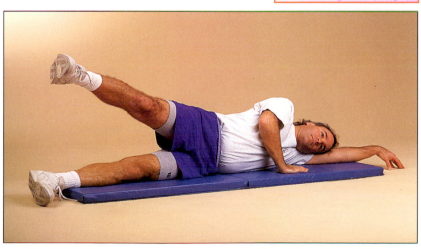

Raise outer leg 16 to 20 inches.

Exercises to Avoid

Deep Knee Bend — strains knees

Jumping Jacks — places strain on outside of knee

Full Sit-Up — not effective in conditioning abdominals

Straight-Leg Sit-Up — may strain lower back

Double Leg Lift — may strain lower back

Donkey Kick — hyperextends back

Bicycle — places stress on neck and back

Squat Thrust — places strain on back and knees

Exercising to Improve Flexibility

Remember that flexibility is the ability to move your joints freely, without pain, through a wide range of motion. This ability requires that the muscles around your joints be stretched safely and regularly. Every group of muscles in your body can be stretched without causing injury to your joints. A safe stretch is one that is gentle and relaxing. You move just until you can feel the muscle stretch. Hold the position for 10 to 20 seconds, then relax and repeat. If a stretch hurts, stop doing it. Pain is a signal from your body that something is wrong. Listen to your body and you'll safely improve your flexibility.

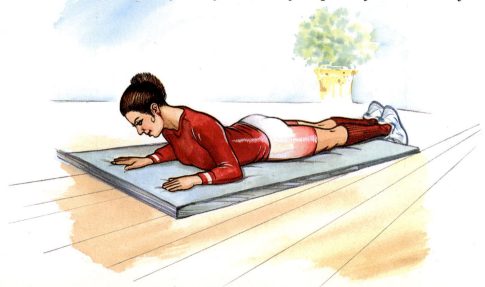

NECK

Head Tilt (Levels 1, 3, 4)

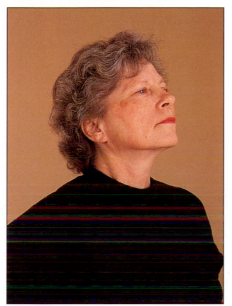

Tilt head back and forth.

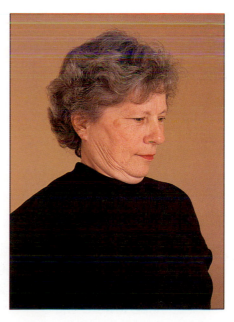

Bend where the head
meets the neck, not
from the lower neck.

Head Turn (Levels 2, 4)

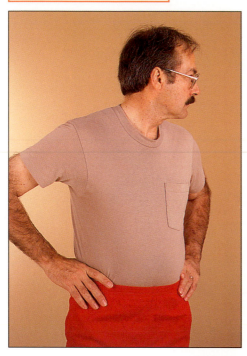

Turn head slowly to look over one shoulder then the other.

Head Lean (Level 3)

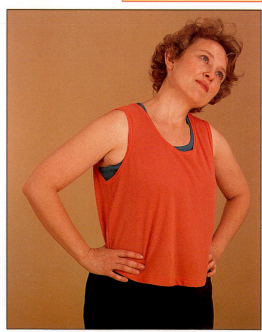

Keep shoulders relaxed; lean head toward one shoulder then the other.

ARMS AND SHOULDERS

Shoulder Rolls (Levels 1, 2, 3, 4)

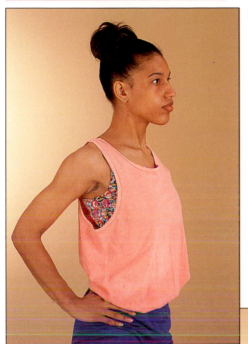

Place hands on hips.

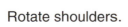

Rotate shoulders.

Shoulder Stretch (Level 2)

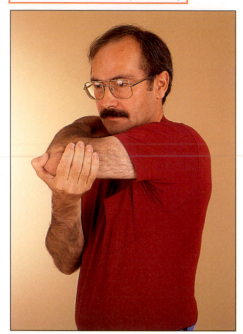

Use right arm to gently pull left elbow across chest, and vice versa.

Arm Circles (Level 3)

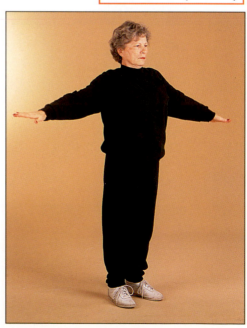

Slowly circle arms from shoulder.

CHEST AND BACK

Standing Cat Stretch (Levels 1, 2, 3, 4)

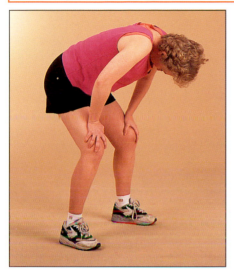

Round then straighten the back while leaning on your thighs.

Chest Stretch (Levels 1, 2, 3, 4)

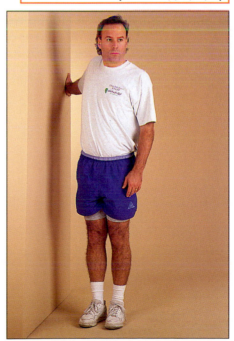

Place outstretched arm against wall, then turn away from the arm.

Side Reach (Levels 1, 2, 4)

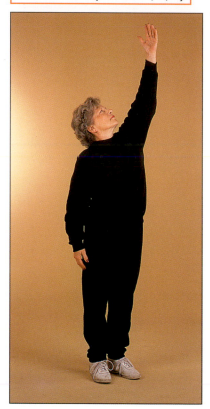

Reach up, not over.

Shoulder Turn (Level 3)

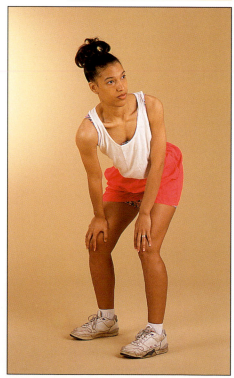

With hands on knees, slowly turn upper body to left, then to right.

Long Lying Stretch (Levels 1, 2, 3, 4)

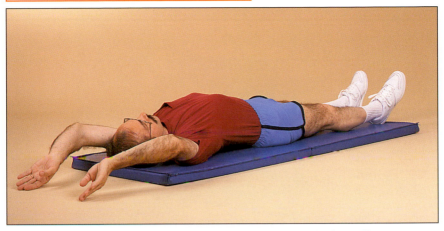

Press lower back to floor as you reach overhead along floor.

Single Knee to Chest (Levels 2, 4)

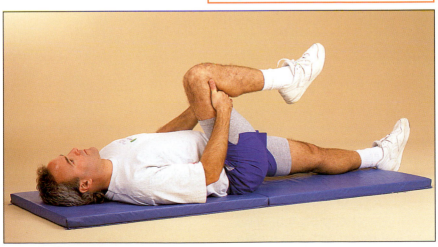

Use both hands placed on back of knee to pull knee toward chest.

Double Knees to Chest (Levels 3, 4)

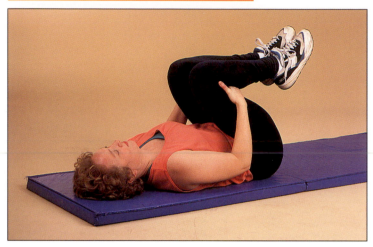

Use both hands placed on backs of knees to pull knees toward chest.

LEGS AND HIPS

Wall Lean (Levels 1, 2, 3, 4)

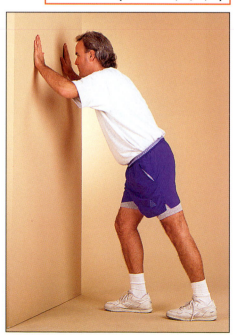

Keep back heel on ground with foot turned slightly inward.

Quadriceps Stretch (Levels 1, 2, 3, 4)

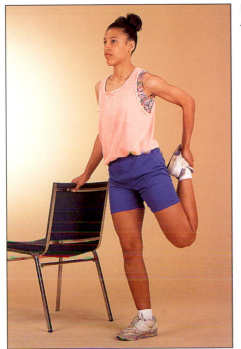

Use hand to bring foot up toward buttocks.

Seated Toe Touch (Levels 1, 2, 3, 4)

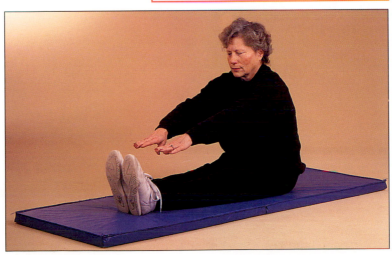

Keep knees bent just a bit.

Standing Lunge (Level 3)

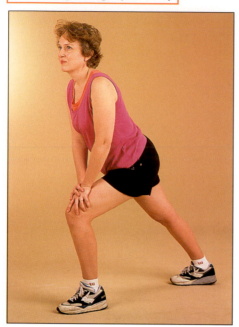

Both feet point forward; front knee is over front toe.

Standing Hamstring Stretch (Level 3)

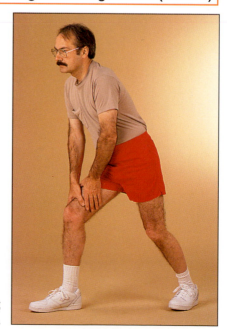

Keep both knees bent slightly; lean over front toe.

ADDITIONAL RECOMMENDED EXERCISES

Triceps Stretch (Arms and Shoulders)

Place your left hand between your shoulder blades.

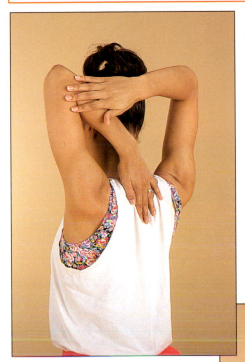

Use your right hand to gently push up and back at your left elbow, then switch sides.

Lying Hamstring Stretch (Legs)

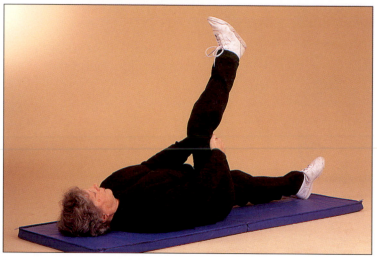

Keep both knees slightly bent as you gently pull one then the other thigh toward your chest.

Elbow Cobra (Back)

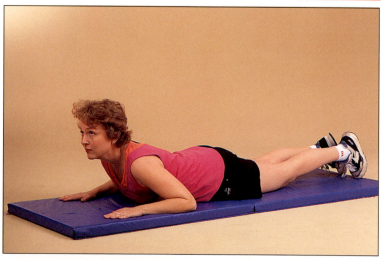

Keep your abdomen on the floor as you lift your upper body.

Butterfly (Legs)

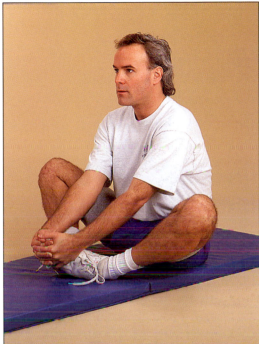

Hold the soles of your feet together.

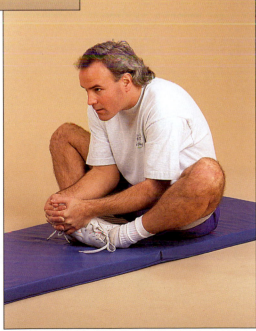

Gently lean forward.

<table>
<tr><td colspan="2">

Exercises to Avoid

Standing Toe Touch — may strain the lower back

Hurdler Stretch — puts strain on bent knee

Hyperextending or Overrounding the Back —puts stress on neck and lower back

Full Neck Circles — hyperextends the neck

Back Bends — ineffective in stretching stomach muscles

</td></tr>
</table>

Exercising to Improve Body Composition

The best way to achieve a healthy body composition is to burn calories through aerobic exercise while using resistance exercise to build lean tissue. If losing body fat is your goal, complete your aerobic fitness program four to six days per week. That, along with a diet low in fat and total calories, will help you to lose the most fat. Most important, make an effort to increase the total amount of activity in your daily life. Keep moving!

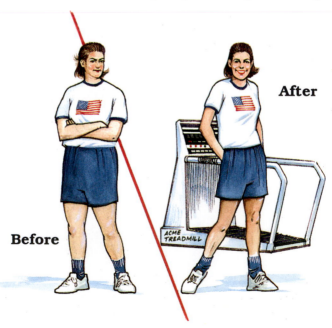

After

Before

ACME TREADMILL

CHAPTER 4

The ACSM Fitness Program

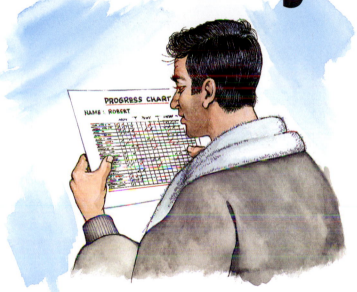

The ACSM Fitness Program is a personalized exercise plan that allows you to work at the correct intensity for your own fitness level. In this chapter, we provide exercises that are appropriate for your fitness in each of the different areas.

How the Program Works

Look at your personal fitness profile on page 25. Like Frank and Jackie, you may be at different fitness levels in each of the fitness areas. In the ACSM Fitness Program, you'll select the exercise level that matches your fitness level for each fitness component. Our color coding makes this easy for you, because the exercise levels in the ACSM Fitness Program match the color coding from the ACSM Fitness Test, as indicated in this chart:

Fitness Test Fitness Level	Color	Fitness Program Exercise Level
Low	Blue	1
Moderate	Green	2
Good	Yellow	3
High	Red	4

Jackie recorded her ACSM Fitness Program results on page 47. Based on their test results, Frank's and Jackie's personal ACSM Fitness Program would include the following:

	Frank	Jackie
Warm-up and aerobic fitness	Level 3	Level 2
Muscular fitness	Level 3	Level 3
Flexibility	Level 1	Level 2
Body composition	Level 3	Level 4

Putting Your Own Program Together

Now, let's plan *your* personal fitness program.

1. Refer to page 25 to check your fitness levels for each fitness component. Indicate each, and the color associated with it, in the table that follows.

Fitness component	Fitness level	Color	Exercise level
Aerobic fitness			
Muscular fitness			
Flexibility			
Body composition			

2. Based on the color code for your fitness level in each of the fitness components, determine the exercise level you should follow for each fitness component (check the chart on page 88), and indicate it in the table. Here's what Jackie's chart looks like:

Fitness component	Fitness level	Color	Exercise level
Aerobic fitness	Below Average	Green	2
Muscular fitness	Average	Yellow	3
Flexibility	Below Average	Green	2
Body composition	Moderate Risk	Red	4

3. Your personal ACSM Fitness Program includes the exercises indicated in each of the four components. Turn to the appropriate sections in the pages at the end of this chapter for lists of the specific exercises you'll be doing. (You can refer back to chapter 3 if you need a reminder of how to do an exercise. We've listed the page number where the photo and description of the exercise appear in chapter 3.)

4. We recommend that you perform the exercises in the order we present them. However, you may find it more enjoyable to rearrange the sequence to fit your personal situation, and that's OK.

5. As you perform the exercises, record your progress in the exercise logs on pages 96–119. Each time you exercise, write the date at the top of a new column. Check off the exercises you perform. It's a good idea to leave yourself little notes about specific exercises. You can write in the margins or, better yet, get a small notebook to record your comments. Frank's muscular fitness program looks like this:

	Week 1				Week 2					Week 3				
Date	8/6	8/7												
Single Arm Row (p. 56)	8 each side				10 each side					12 each side				
	✔	✔												
Stair Stepping (p. 61)	8 each side				10 each side					12 each side				
	✔	✔												
Straight Arm Curl-Up (p. 65)	8 times				10 times					12 times				
	✔	✔												
Knee Push-Up (p. 55)	6 times				8 times					11 times				
	✔	✔												
Prone Single Leg Lift (p. 66)	6 each side				8 each side					11 each side				
	✔	✔												

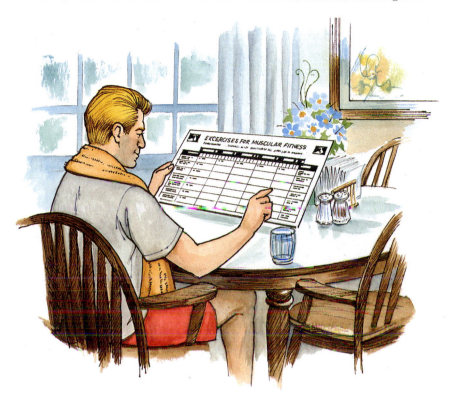

6. Progress to a new time or number of repetitions only when you can complete the time or number indicated. You may continue to progress in the other exercises even if you must stay back in a particular exercise for several days. This way, you'll be able to tailor your exercise program to your individual rate of progress. When you reach the end of week 6, continue with all exercises in the program until all exercises have caught up to the same level.

7. Once you've reached the end of your six-week program, it's time to reassess your fitness levels. Chapter 5 provides information on how to use your reassessment information.

Exercising Safely and Wisely

As we explained in chapter 2, exercise is safe for most adults. There are, however, things you can do both to ensure your safety while exercising and to maximize the health benefits you'll derive.

Drink extra water.

Drink a cup of water before you exercise and another after. Drink an additional cup of water every 15 to 20 minutes during exercise. Carry a water bottle with you during your aerobic exercise.

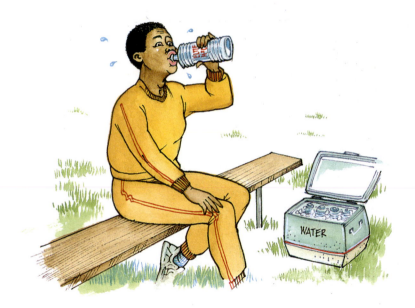

Increase the percentage of your calories that come from carbohydrates, fruits, and vegetables.

Eat more carbohydrates in foods such as bread, pasta, rice, and potatoes, as well as fruits and vegetables, while decreasing the amounts of fatty foods such as meat, butter, and desserts. Carbohydrates are a major fuel source for exercise, and as you sweat, you lose minerals, which fruits and vegetables can replace.

You don't need to take any extra vitamins or other supplements when exercising.

A well-balanced diet provides all of the nutrients a healthy, active person needs. Despite what many supplement manufacturers and "health" food stores would like you to believe, additional vitamins, proteins, amino acids, or other products are not necessary, and they won't improve your performance.

Follow your doctor's recommendations concerning any medications you may be taking.

If you're on a medically supervised diet, you can still participate in the ACSM Fitness Program. The exercises may increase your weight loss in addition to increasing your fitness.

Pay attention to any discomfort you may feel during exercise.

It's normal to feel a bit stiff or sore a day or two after beginning your exercise program. This stiffness or pain should disappear in a few days. However, if you experience sudden pain while performing any of the exercises listed in your program, stop that exercise and go on to the next. During your next exercise session, try all the exercises again. If you still have pain or discomfort while doing a particular exercise, especially it it's in the upper body or chest, stop doing it until you consult with your doctor about it during your next physical exam.

Adjust your exercise when you aren't feeling well.

When you're sick, your body needs its resources to fight off the illness. Be kind to yourself, and take a few days off from your exercise program.

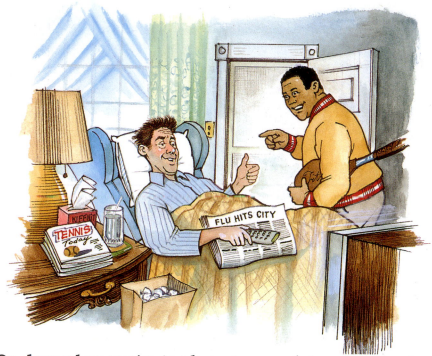

On days when you're too busy to complete your exercise program, complete whatever portion you can, even if it's only 10 or 15 minutes.

However, on such days, try to deliberately increase activity throughout the day. Remember that all appropriate physical activity contributes to your overall health.

Don't worry if you must miss a workout. Missing an occasional workout won't affect your fitness.

But, after missing workouts for two weeks, you may begin to see a decline in your fitness. You may want to restart your exercise program using the exercises you had already completed one week before you began missing your workouts. After three to five months of missed workouts, you may have lost all the fitness improvement you gained. If you must miss your workouts for extended periods, we suggest that you reassess your fitness status to see if you need to adjust your program.

Adjust your exercise based on the weather.

Sometimes the weather doesn't cooperate, and you can't perform your usual activity. At such times, try to find alternate exercise opportunities, such as walking at malls or using that exercise bike in the basement. Sometimes the weather affords new opportunities for exercise. Take advantage of special opportunities such as hiking or cross-country skiing to vary your exercise program.

ACSM Fitness Programs and Logs

Now it's time to start using all the information you've put together to begin your own ACSM Fitness Program. Everything you need to use the program is included on these program log sheets. You'll find the exercises you need to do (along with the page number in chapter 3 where each is described), the time or suggested number of repetitions for each exercise, and a place to record whether you've completed the exercise. Don't forget to warm up before you begin. Remember that body composition improves as you do aerobic and resistance exercises. The number of times you exercise each week is a good way to evaluate whether your program will contribute to a healthy body composition.

Exercises for Warm–Up and Aerobic Fitness

Equipment: Stopwatch or watch with a second hand

	Week 1	Week 2	Week 3
Date			
Shoulder Rolls (p. 75)	3 backward, 3 forward	3 backward, 3 forward	3 backward, 3 forward
Head Tilt (p. 73)	10 sec. 2 times	10 sec. 2 times	10 sec. 2 times
Walk in Place	2 min	2 min	2 min
Side Reach (p. 78)	5 each side	5 each side	5 each side
Standing Cat Stretch (p. 77)	10 sec. 2 times	10 sec. 2 times	10 sec. 2 times
Chest Stretch (p. 77)	10 sec . each side	10 sec. each side	10 sec. each side
Wall Lean (p. 80)	10 sec. each side	10 sec. each side	10 sec. each side
Quadriceps Stretch (p. 81)	10 sec. each side	10 sec. each side	10 sec. each side
Walking	10 min: 5 out and back	12 min: 6 out and back	15 min: 7:30 out and back

LEVEL 1

Week 4	Week 5	Week 6	Date
3 backward, 3 forward	3 backward, 3 forward	3 backward, 3 forward	**Shoulder Rolls (p. 75)**
10 sec. 2 times	10 sec. 2 times	10 sec. 2 times	**Head Tilt (p. 73)**
2 min	2 min	2 min	**Walk in Place**
7 each side	8 each side	10 each side	**Side Reach (p. 78)**
15 sec. 2 times	15 sec. 2 times	15 sec. 2 times	**Standing Cat Stretch (p. 77)**
15 sec. each side	15 sec. each side	15 sec. each side	**Chest Stretch (p. 77)**
15 sec. each side	15 sec. each side	15 sec. each side	**Wall Lean (p. 80)**
15 sec. each side	15 sec. each side	15 sec. each side	**Quadriceps Stretch (p. 81)**
15 min: 8 out, 7 back (Walk faster back.)	20 min: 10 out, 10 back	20 min: 10 out, 10 back (Walk farther each day.)	**Walking**

Exercises for Warm–Up and Aerobic Fitness

Equipment: Stopwatch or watch with a second hand

LEVEL 2

	Week 1	Week 2	Week 3
Date			
Shoulder Rolls (p. 75)	5 backward, 5 forward	5 backward, 5 forward	5 backward, 5 forward
Head Turn (p. 74)	5 sec. each side 2 times	5 sec. each side 2 times	5 sec. each side 2 times
Walk in Place	2 min	2 min	2 min
Side Reach (p. 78)	10 each side	10 each side	10 each side
Standing Cat Stretch (p. 77)	15 sec. 2 times	15 sec. 2 times	15 sec. 2 times
Chest Stretch (p. 77)	15 sec. each side	15 sec. each side	15 sec. each side
Shoulder Stretch (p. 76)	15 sec. each side	15 sec. each side	15 sec. each side
Wall Lean (p. 80)	15 sec. each side	15 sec. each side	15 sec. each side
Seated Toe Touch (p. 81)	15 sec. 2 times	15 sec. 2 times	15 sec. 2 times
Walking	20 min: 10 out, 10 back	20 min: 10 out, 10 back (Walk farther each day.)	25 min: 12:30 out and back

LEVEL 2

Week 4	Week 5	Week 6	Date
5 backward, 5 forward	5 backward, 5 forward	5 backward, 5 forward	**Shoulder Rolls (p. 75)**
10 sec. each side 2 times	10 sec. each side 2 times	10 sec. each side 2 times	**Head Turn (p. 74)**
2 min	2 min	2 min	**Walk in Place**
12 each side	13 each side	15 each side	**Side Reach (p. 78)**
15 sec. 3 times	15 sec. 3 times	15 sec. 3 times	**Standing Cat Stretch (p. 77)**
20 sec. each side	20 sec. each side	20 sec. each side	**Chest Stretch (p. 77)**
20 sec. each side	20 sec. each side	20 sec. each side	**Shoulder Stretch (p. 76)**
20 sec. each side	20 sec. each side	20 sec. each side	**Wall Lean (p. 80)**
20 sec. 2 times	20 sec. 2 times	20 sec. 2 times	**Seated Toe Touch (p. 81)**
25 min: 13 out, 12 back (Walk faster back.)	30 min: 15 out and back	30 min: 15 out and back (Walk farther each day.)	**Walking**

Exercises for
Warm–Up and Aerobic Fitness

Equipment: Stopwatch or watch with a second hand

	Week 1	Week 2	Week 3
Date			
Head Tilt (p. 73)	10 sec. 2 times	10 sec. 2 times	10 sec. 2 times
Head Lean (p. 74)	10 sec. each side	10 sec. each side	10 sec. each side
Walk in Place	2 min	2 min	2 min
Arm Circles (p. 76)	5 forward, 5 backward	5 forward, 5 backward	5 forward, 5 backward
Standing Cat Stretch (p. 77)	15 sec. 3 times	15 sec. 3 times	15 sec. 3 times
Shoulder Turn (p. 78)	15 sec. each side	15 sec. each side	15 sec. each side
Chest Stretch (p. 77)	20 sec. each side	20 sec. each side	20 sec. each side
Standing Lunge (p. 82)	15 sec. each side	15 sec. each side	15 sec. each side
Standing Hamstring Stretch (p. 82)	15 sec. each side	15 sec. each side	15 sec. each side
Walking	30 min: 15 out and back	30 min: 15 out and back (Walk farther each day.)	35 min: 17:30 out and back

LEVEL 3

Week 4	Week 5	Week 6	Date
10 sec. 2 times	10 sec. 2 times	10 sec. 2 times	**Head Tilt** **(p. 73)**
10 sec. each side	10 sec. each side	10 sec. each side	**Head Lean** **(p. 74)**
2 min	2 min	2 min	**Walk in Place**
7 forward, 7 backward	8 forward, 8 backward	10 forward, 10 backward	**Arm Circles** **(p. 76)**
15 sec. 3 times	15 sec. 3 times	15 sec. 3 times	**Standing Cat** **Stretch (p. 77)**
20 sec. each side	20 sec. each side	20 sec. each side	**Shoulder Turn** **(p. 78)**
20 sec. each side	20 sec. each side	20 sec. each side	**Chest Stretch** **(p. 77)**
20 sec. each side	20 sec. each side	20 sec. each side	**Standing Lunge** **(p. 82)**
20 sec. each side	20 sec. each side	20 sec. each side	**Standing** **Hamstring** **Stretch (p. 82)**
35 min: 18 out, 17 back (Walk faster back.)	40 min: 20 out and back	40 min: 20 out and back (Walk farther each day.)	**Walking**

Exercises for
Warm-Up and Aerobic Fitness

Equipment: Stopwatch or watch with a
second hand

	Week 1	Week 2	Week 3
Date			
Shoulder Rolls (p. 75)	5 backward, 5 forward	5 backward, 5 forward	5 backward, 5 forward
Head Tilt (p. 73)	10 sec. 2 times	10 sec. 2 times	10 sec. 2 times
Head Turn (p. 74)	10 sec. each side, 2 times	10 sec. each side, 2 times	10 sec. each side, 2 times
Walk in Place	2 min	2 min	2 min
Side Reach (p. 78)	5 each side	5 each side	5 each side
Standing Cat Stretch (p. 77)	10 sec. 2 times	10 sec. 2 times	10 sec. 2 times
Chest Stretch (p. 77)	10 sec. each side	10 sec. each side	10 sec. each side
Wall Lean (p. 80)	10 sec. each side	10 sec. each side	10 sec. each side
Quadriceps Stretch (p. 81)	10 sec. each side	10 sec. each side	10 sec. each side
Walking	40 min: 20 out and back	40 min: 20 out and back (Walk farther each day.)	40 min: 20:30 out, 19:30 back (Walk faster back.)

LEVEL 4

Week 4	Week 5	Week 6	Date
5 backward, 5 forward	5 backward, 5 forward	5 backward, 5 forward	**Shoulder Rolls (p. 75)**
10 sec. 2 times	10 sec. 2 times	10 sec. 2 times	**Head Tilt (p. 73)**
10 sec. each side, 2 times	10 sec. each side, 2 times	10 sec. each side, 2 times	**Head Turn (p. 74)**
2 min	2 min	2 min	**Walk in Place**
7 each side	7 each side	7 each side	**Side Reach (p. 78)**
15 sec. 2 times	15 sec. 2 times	15 sec. 2 times	**Standing Cat Stretch (p. 77)**
15 sec. each side	15 sec. each side	15 sec. each side	**Chest Stretch (p. 77)**
15 sec. each side	15 sec. each side	15 sec. each side	**Wall Lean (p. 80)**
15 sec. each side	15 sec. each side	15 sec. each side	**Quadriceps Stretch (p. 81)**
45 min: 22:30 out and back	45 min: 23 out, 22 back (Walk faster back.)	45 min: Find a pleasant loop, rather than an out and back path.	**Walking**

LEVEL 1

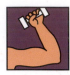

Exercises for
Muscular Fitness

Equipment: A sturdy chair; Plastic jugs partially
filled with water or sand.

Date	Week 1			Week 2			Week 3		
Wall Push-Up (p. 53)	4 times			6 times			8 times		
Single Arm Row (p. 56)	4 each side			6 each side			8 each side		
Seated Lower Leg Lift (p. 59)	4 each side			6 each side			8 each side		
Neck Curl-Up (p. 64)	4 times			6 times			8 times		

Week 4	Week 5	Week 6	Date
11 times	13 times	15 times	**Wall Push-Up (p. 53)**
11 each side	13 each side	15 each side	**Single Arm Row (p. 56)**
11 each side	13 each side	15 each side	**Seated Lower Leg Lift (p. 59)**
11 times	13 times	15 times	**Neck Curl-Up (p. 64)**

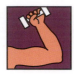

Exercises for Muscular Fitness

Equipment: A sturdy chair; Plastic jugs partially filled with water or sand.

Date	Week 1	Week 2	Week 3
Chair Push-Up (p. 54)	4 times	5 times	6 times
Toe Raise - use a chair (p. 63)	4 times	5 times	6 times
Seated Straight Leg Lift (p. 60)	6 each side	8 each side	11 each side
Single Arm Row (p. 56)	6 each side	8 each side	11 each side
Shoulder Curl-Up (p. 64)	6 times	8 times	11 times
Prone Neck Lift (p. 66)	4 times	5 times	6 times

LEVEL 2

LEVEL 2

Week 4	Week 5	Week 6	Date
8 times	11 times	15 times	**Chair Push-Up (p. 54)**
8 times	11 times	15 times	**Toe Raise - use a chair (p. 63)**
14 each side	17 each side	20 each side	**Seated Straight Leg Lift (p. 60)**
14 each side	17 each side	20 each side	**Single Arm Row (p. 56)**
14 times	17 times	20 times	**Shoulder Curl-Up (p. 64)**
8 times	11 times	15 times	**Prone Neck Lift (p. 66)**

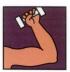

Exercises for Muscular Fitness

Equipment: A bench or step 8 to 12 inches high; Plastic jugs partially filled with water or sand.

	Week 1				Week 2				Week 3			
Date												
Single Arm Row (p. 56)	8 each side				10 each side				12 each side			
Stair Stepping (p. 61)	8 each side				10 each side				12 each side			
Straight Arm Curl-Up (p. 65)	8 times				10 times				12 times			
Knee Push-Up (p. 55)	6 times				8 times				11 times			
Prone Single Leg Lift (p. 66)	6 each side				8 each side				11 each side			

LEVEL 3

Week 4	Week 5	Week 6	Date
14 each side	17 each side	20 each side	**Single Arm Row (p. 56)**
14 each side	17 each side	20 each side	**Stair Stepping (p. 61)**
14 times	17 times	20 times	**Straight Arm Curl-Up (p. 65)**
14 times	17 times	20 times	**Knee Push-Up (p. 55)**
14 each side	17 each side	20 each side	**Prone Single Leg Lift (p. 66)**

LEVEL 4

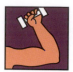

Exercises for Muscular Fitness

Equipment: A sturdy chair; Plastic jugs partially filled with water or sand.

	Week 1		Week 2		Week 3	
Date						
Biceps Curl (p. 57)	6 each side		8 each side		11 each side	
Reverse Fly (p. 58)	6 each side		8 each side		11 each side	
Chair Squat (p. 62)	6 times		8 times		11 times	
Toe Raise - Use a chair (p. 63)	6 each side		8 each side		11 each side	
Toe Push-Up (p. 55)	6 times		8 times		11 times	
Prone Head and Leg Lift (p. 67)	6 each side		8 each side		11 each side	
Crossed-Arm Curl-Up (p. 65)	8 times		10 times		12 times	

Week 4	Week 5	Week 6	Date
14 each side	17 each side	20 each side	**Biceps Curl (p. 57)**
14 each side	17 each side	20 each side	**Reverse Fly (p. 58)**
14 times	17 times	20 times	**Chair Squat (p. 62)**
14 each side	17 each side	20 each side	**Toe Raise - Use a chair (p. 63)**
14 times	17 times	20 times	**Toe Push-Up (p. 55)**
14 each side	17 each side	20 each side	**Prone Head and Leg Lift (p. 67)**
14 times	17 times	20 times	**Crossed-Arm Curl-Up (p. 65)**

Exercises for Flexibility and Cool–Down

Equipment: Watch or clock with a second hand

Date	Week 1			Week 2			Week 3		
Shoulder Rolls (p. 75)	3 backward, 3 forward			3 backward, 3 forward			3 backward, 3 forward		
Chest Stretch (p. 77)	10 sec. each side 2 times			10 sec. each side 2 times			15 sec. each side 2 times		
Wall Lean (p. 80)	10 sec. each side 2 times			10 sec. each side 2 times			15 sec. each side 2 times		
Quadriceps Stretch (p. 81)	10 sec. each side 2 times			10 sec. each side 2 times			15 sec. each side 2 times		
Seated Toe-Touch (p. 81)	10 sec. 2 times			10 sec. 2 times			15 sec. 2 times		
Long Lying Stretch (p. 79)	10 sec. 2 times			10 sec. 2 times			10 sec. 2 times		

LEVEL 1

Week 4	Week 5	Week 6	Date
3 backward, 3 forward	3 backward, 3 forward	3 backward, 3 forward	**Shoulder Rolls (p. 75)**
15 sec. each side 2 times	20 sec. each side 2 times	20 sec. each side 2 times	**Chest Stretch (p. 77)**
15 sec. each side 2 times	20 sec. each side 2 times	20 sec. each side 2 times	**Wall Lean (p. 80)**
15 sec. each side 2 times	20 sec. each side 2 times	20 sec. each side 2 times	**Quadriceps Stretch (p. 81)**
15 sec. 2 times	20 sec. 2 times	20 sec. 2 times	**Seated Toe-Touch (p. 81)**
10 sec. 2 times	10 sec. 2 times	10 sec. 2 times	**Long Lying Stretch (p. 79)**

Exercises for Flexibility and Cool–Down

Equipment: Watch or clock with a second hand

Date	Week 1	Week 2	Week 3
Shoulder Rolls (p. 75)	5 backward, 5 forward	5 backward, 5 forward	5 backward, 5 forward
Chest Stretch (p. 77)	20 sec. each side 2 times	20 sec. each side 2 times	20 sec. each side 2 times
Wall Lean (p. 80)	20 sec. each side 2 times	20 sec. each side 2 times	20 sec. each side 2 times
Quadriceps Stretch (p. 81)	20 sec. each side 2 times	20 sec. each side 2 times	20 sec. each side 2 times
Seated Toe-Touch (p. 81)	20 sec. 2 times	20 sec. 2 times	20 sec. 2 times
Single Knee to Chest (p. 79)	10 sec. each side 2 times	10 sec. each side 2 times	15 sec. each side 2 times
Long Lying Stretch (p. 79)	15 sec. 2 times	15 sec. 2 times	15 sec. 2 times

LEVEL 2

Week 4	Week 5	Week 6	Date
5 backward, 5 forward	5 backward, 5 forward	5 backward, 5 forward	**Shoulder Rolls (p. 75)**
20 sec. each side 2 times	20 sec. each side 2 times	20 sec. each side 2 times	**Chest Stretch (p. 77)**
20 sec. each side 2 times	20 sec. each side 2 times	20 sec. each side 2 times	**Wall Lean (p. 80)**
20 sec. each side 2 times	20 sec. each side 2 times	20 sec. each side 2 times	**Quadriceps Stretch (p. 81)**
20 sec. 2 times	20 sec. 2 times	20 sec. 2 times	**Seated Toe-Touch (p. 81)**
15 sec. each side 2 times	20 sec. each side 2 times	20 sec. each side 2 times	**Single Knee to Chest (p. 79)**
15 sec. 2 times	15 sec. 2 times	15 sec. 2 times	**Long Lying Stretch (p. 79)**

Exercises for Flexibility and Cool–Down

Equipment: Watch or clock with a second hand

	Week 1	Week 2	Week 3
Date			
Shoulder Rolls (p. 75)	5 backward, 5 forward	5 backward, 5 forward	5 backward, 5 forward
Chest Stretch (p. 77)	20 sec. each side 2 times	20 sec. each side 2 times	20 sec. each side 2 times
Wall Lean (p. 80)	20 sec. each side 2 times	20 sec. each side 2 times	20 sec. each side 2 times
Quadriceps Stretch (p. 81)	20 sec. each side 2 times	20 sec. each side 2 times	20 sec. each side 2 times
Seated Toe-Touch (p. 81)	20 sec. 2 times	20 sec. 2 times	20 sec. 2 times
Double Knees to Chest (p. 80)	10 sec. each side 2 times	10 sec. each side 2 times	15 sec. each side 2 times
Long Lying Stretch (p. 79)	15 sec. 2 times	15 sec. 2 times	15 sec. 2 times

LEVEL 3

LEVEL 3

Week 4	Week 5	Week 6	Date
5 backward, 5 forward	5 backward, 5 forward	5 backward, 5 forward	**Shoulder Rolls (p. 75)**
20 sec. each side 2 times	20 sec. each side 2 times	20 sec. each side 2 times	**Chest Stretch (p. 77)**
20 sec. each side 2 times	20 sec. each side 2 times	20 sec. each side 2 times	**Wall Lean (p. 80)**
20 sec. each side 2 times	20 sec. each side 2 times	20 sec. each side 2 times	**Quadriceps Stretch (p. 81)**
20 sec. 2 times	20 sec. 2 times	20 sec. 2 times	**Seated Toe-Touch (p. 81)**
15 sec. each side 2 times	20 sec. each side 2 times	20 sec. each side 2 times	**Double Knees to Chest (p. 80)**
15 sec. 2 times	15 sec. 2 times	15 sec. 2 times	**Long Lying Stretch (p. 79)**

Exercises for Flexibility and Cool–Down

Equipment: Watch or clock with a second hand

	Week 1	Week 2	Week 3
Date			
Shoulder Rolls (p. 75)	5 backward, 5 forward	5 backward, 5 forward	5 backward, 5 forward
Chest Stretch (p. 77)	20 sec. each side 2 times	20 sec. each side 2 times	20 sec. each side 2 times
Wall Lean (p. 80)	20 sec. each side 2 times	20 sec. each side 2 times	20 sec. each side 2 times
Quadriceps Stretch (p. 81)	20 sec. each side 2 times	20 sec. each side 2 times	20 sec. each side 2 times
Seated Toe-Touch (p. 81)	20 sec. 2 times	20 sec. 2 times	20 sec. 2 times
Single Knee to Chest (p. 79)	10 sec. each side 2 times	10 sec. each side 2 times	15 sec. each side 2 times
Double Knees to Chest (p. 80)	10 sec. each side 2 times	10 sec. each side 2 times	15 sec. each side 2 times
Long Lying Stretch (p. 79)	15 sec. 2 times	15 sec. 2 times	15 sec. 2 times

LEVEL 4

LEVEL 4

Week 4	Week 5	Week 6	Date
5 backward, 5 forward	5 backward, 5 forward	5 backward, 5 forward	**Shoulder Rolls (p. 75)**
20 sec. each side 2 times	20 sec. each side 2 times	20 sec. each side 2 times	**Chest Stretch (p. 77)**
20 sec. each side 2 times	20 sec. each side 2 times	20 sec. each side 2 times	**Wall Lean (p. 80)**
20 sec. each side 2 times	20 sec. each side 2 times	20 sec. each side 2 times	**Quadriceps Stretch (p. 81)**
20 sec. 2 times	20 sec. 2 times	20 sec. 2 times	**Seated Toe-Touch (p. 81)**
15 sec. each side 2 times	20 sec. each side 2 times	20 sec. each side 2 times	**Single Knee to Chest (p. 79)**
15 sec. each side 2 times	20 sec. each side 2 times	20 sec. each side 2 times	**Double Knees to Chest (p. 80)**
15 sec. 2 times	15 sec. 2 times	15 sec. 2 times	**Long Lying Stretch (p. 79)**

Recommended Frequencies of Exercise Based on Body Composition Assessments

Level 1 - Blue

Your body composition assessments indicate that the amount of body fat you have *may* be too low. We recommend that you consult your doctor before beginning an exercise program.

Level 2 - Green

Your body composition assessments indicate that the amount of body fat you have *may* be too high. We recommend that you exercise four to six days per week for aerobic fitness, at least three days per week for flexibility, and two to three days per week for muscular fitness.

Level 3 - Yellow

Your body composition assessments indicate that the amount of body fat you have is moderate. We recommend that you do aerobic and flexibility exercises three to five days a week and muscular fitness exercises two to three days per week.

Level 4 - Red

Your body composition assessments indicate that the amount of body fat you have is good. We recommend that you do aerobic and flexibility exercises three to five days per week, and muscular fitness exercises two to three days per week.

CHAPTER 5

The Next Step

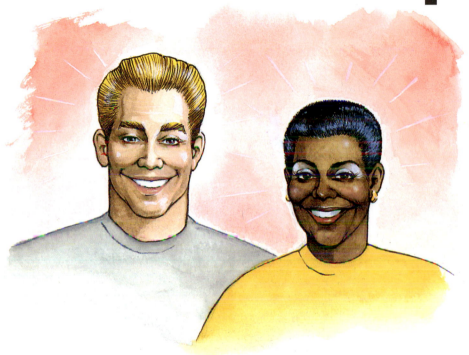

Frank and Jackie are thrilled to have completed the exercises for the first six weeks of each fitness component. They're already noticing that they have more energy. If you've also finished one level of the ACSM Fitness Program, it's time to reassess your current fitness status and reevaluate your goals. Go back and do the assessments in the ACSM Fitness Test again (in chapter 2). Then review the fitness goals you identified on page 16. Your fitness test results will show how you've progressed toward your goals.

Jackie has met her first goal of being able to walk three miles without stopping, but she's not quite at her body mass index goal. Frank feels good about being able to reach seven inches in the sit-and-reach test, which shows his flexibility is improving. Are you moving toward your goals? Do you have new goals for your personal fitness program? If your goals continue to indicate that you'd like to improve your fitness in one or more areas, then use the results of your updated assessment as a guide to selecting your new exercise level in each of the fitness components of the ACSM Fitness Program. Many of the exercises will be familiar to you, but you'll also notice some new exercises.

After you've completed all of the levels in the ACSM Fitness Program, or when you are ready for something different, this chapter can help you take the next step in your personal fitness program. Perhaps you'd like to add new activities to your fitness program or to join a fitness center. This chapter provides you with information on how to continue your active lifestyle.

Increasing Daily Physical Activity

Ample scientific evidence shows clearly that participation in a structured exercise program will help you maintain your health. However, when you can't be involved in such a program, maintaining adequate amounts of physical activity through your daily tasks is essential. The risk of developing chronic diseases such as diabetes, heart disease, and cancer are decreased for people who engage in regular physical activity. You can increase daily activity in many ways, including these:

- Walking rather than driving to complete short errands
- Deliberately parking farther from an entrance than you need to
- Leaving home a few minutes early to allow yourself time for a short walk before work
- Taking a short walk during coffee breaks or lunch

- Using stairs rather than elevators or escalators for short climbs
- Doing your own lawn work, gardening, or housework
- Carrying a few packages to your car rather than using the shopping cart
- Walking your pet
- Scheduling play time with your children or grandchildren
- Walking rather than using a cart on the golf course

Activities to Improve Cardiorespiratory Endurance

Walking is not the only exercise that will improve your cardio-respiratory endurance. Other activities that use large muscle groups in a continuous, rhythmic fashion will give you similar results. Here are some good aerobic activities, along with approximately how many calories they require during 30 minutes of exercise:

Activity	Calories used in 30 minutes	
	140 lb person	180 lb person
Bicycling, 10 mph	200	260
Cross-country skiing	260	350
Dancing – aerobic, moderate	200	260
Dancing – ballroom, leisure	130	170
Hiking	160	200
Ice skating, moderate	230	300
In-line skating	230	300
Jogging, 12 min per mile	260	350
Riding machine	180	220
Rope skipping, 80 per min	330	430
Rowing, moderate	230	300
Stair climbing	260	350
Swimming – freestyle, moderate	260	350

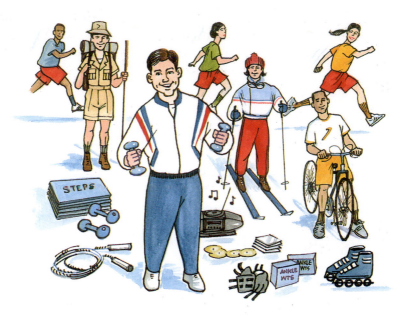

You can do any of these activities, or a mixture of them, throughout the week. To improve your cardiorespiratory endurance you simply need to do some form of aerobic activity at least three days a week. Remember that to maintain good health it is most important to stay active, whatever form that activity may take. Staying active is one of the most important things you can do for your health.

Guidelines for Healthy Aerobic Activity

- Exercise three to five times per week.
- Warm up for 5 to 10 minutes before aerobic activity.
- Maintain your exercise intensity for 30 to 45 minutes.
- Gradually decrease the intensity, then stretch to cool down during the last 5 to 10 minutes.
- If weight loss is a major goal, participate in your aerobic activity *at least* 30 minutes, five days per week.

On days when you can't complete your exercise program, complete whatever portion you can, even if it's only 10 or 15 minutes. Additionally, deliberately increase activity throughout the day. Remember that all appropriate physical activity contributes to your overall health.

Choosing Activities for Aerobic Exercise

You should consider several factors when choosing an aerobic activity for your personal fitness program.

Impact

Some aerobic activities, such as skipping rope, running, and high-impact aerobics, involve jumping and pounding that may be uncomfortable or lead to injury. Swimming, cross-country skiing, in-line skating, cycling, and rowing are easier on the joints.

Convenience

Some aerobic activities require expensive equipment, are seasonal, or are not readily available in certain locations. For example, it's hard to make cross-country skiing a regular part of your fitness routine if it never snows where you live.

Skill

Activities that require a lot of skill may discourage you. It takes a while to learn to use in-line skates, for example. Many people quit exercising before they've developed the skills they need for the activity to become enjoyable.

Social factors

Exercising with a group can be fun and beneficial. Sometimes, exercising with other people is such fun that you're more likely to continue with your fitness program than if you try to exercise alone. At other times, exercising by yourself allows you to complete your exercise program at your own pace without being viewed or judged by others. Most aerobic activities can be done alone or with a group, while others, for safety reasons, are best done with a group.

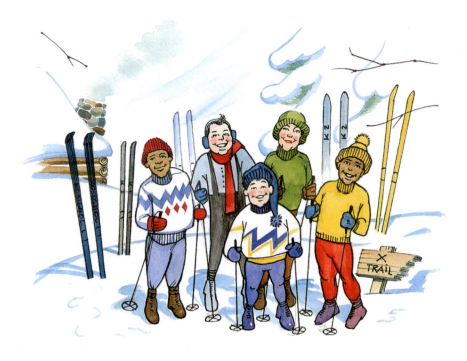

Enjoyment

Because increasing the amount of physical activity in your daily life is so important to your health, it's essential that you choose one or several activities that you really enjoy. Even if the activities you choose don't seem to provide as "hard" a workout as other activities, you're more likely to continue exercising when you enjoy what you're doing. Selecting more than one activity and rotating the activities regularly will help prevent boredom and increase the likelihood of your continuing to exercise.

Choosing the Intensity of Aerobic Exercise

A good way to determine if you're working hard enough during your aerobic exercise is to measure your heart rate. First, calculate your *exercise heart rate range* using the steps in the box below. Then, during your exercise, find your pulse at one of the places described on page 26. If your heart rate is within the range you've calculated, your pace is good! For example, Frank's estimated maximum heart rate is 183 beats per minute (220 – 37). By multiplying 183 by 0.6 and by 0.9, Frank determines that his exercise heart rate range is between 110 and 165 beats per minute. Jackie's exercise heart rate range is between 103 and 155 beats per minute.

Calculating Your Exercise Heart Rate Range

1. Estimate your maximum heart rate.

   220 – age = _____ (maximum heart rate)

2. Determine your lower-limit exercise heart rate by multiplying your maximum heart rate by 0.6.

   maximum heart rate _____ × 0.6 = _____

3. Determine your upper-limit exercise heart rate by multiplying your maximum heart rate by 0.9.

   maximum heart rate _____ × 0.9 = _____

4. Your *exercise heart rate range* is between your upper and lower limits

   Note: Medications for high blood pressure or other conditions may affect your heart rate during exercise. Therefore, if you are taking such medications, consult your physician before determining your exercise heart rate range.

For most people, exercising at the lower end of the exercise heart rate range for a longer time is better than exercising at the higher end of the range for a shorter time. Exercising at lower intensity will improve your fitness, and it offers several advantages over higher-intensity exercise:

- You decrease your risk of orthopedic problems.
- Your risk of cardiovascular complications is lower.
- You are more likely to continue your fitness program over a long time.

Activities for Muscular Strength and Endurance

Progressing in your muscular strength and endurance program can be as simple as continuing to do the exercises in the ACSM Fitness Program, but with heavier weights or more repetitions. Additionally, you may want to join a fitness center or purchase home weight-training equipment. Regardless of the method you choose to progress in your program, follow these guidelines to ensure safe, effective exercise:

Guidelines for Muscular Strength and Endurance Activities

- Include exercises for each of the muscle areas shown in chapter 3.
- Complete 8 to 15 repetitions of each exercise. When you can easily complete 15 repetitions, increase the workload in either, or both, of these ways:
  — Increase the amount of weight you lift.
  — Do a second set of 8 to 15 repetitions.

Commercial Fitness Facilities and Equipment

If you are ready for some additional variety in your exercise program, many opportunities are open to you. Most communities have fitness centers, and stores are filled with exercise equipment, videos, and books. This section helps you select the best ones for you.

General Guidelines for Selecting Exercise Equipment for Home Use

You may choose to expand your home exercise program by purchasing aerobic exercise or weight-training equipment.

Exercising at home saves both the time and expense of fitness center membership. It also allows you to exercise in privacy.

Choosing the best equipment and programs may seem complicated—and expensive! Many different types of exercise equipment and programs are available for use in your home. Choices range from $20 collapsible equipment or videos to $10,000 state-of-the-art models. To add to the confusion, not all advertised products actually produce the desired results. If an advertiser's claim sounds too good to be true, it probably is!

Products to Avoid

If a product makes any of the following claims, avoid it. No exercise program or equipment can safely produce these claimed results.

• "You'll see results immediately!" Real improvements in your fitness take time. You may see some changes in just a few days or weeks. Other changes may take a bit longer. By regularly assessing your fitness using the ACSM Fitness Test, you'll have a good indication of your personal progress.

• "An effortless, no-sweat workout!" If getting fit took no effort, everyone would be fit! It takes effort and self-determination to improve your fitness. The ACSM Fitness Program is designed to help make your efforts more productive.

• "Lose fat from your thighs (or waist, or wherever); rid yourself of that cellulite!" No exercise reduces fat specifically in the area exercised. During exercise, the body takes its energy from the fat stored all over your body. Cellulite is simply a name given to the dimpled fat that tends to accumulate on women's hips and thighs and on men's abdomens. Appropriate aerobic exercise will help reduce overall body fat and hence the "cellulite" appearance.

• "Wear this special clothing (or vest or belt) and lose inches off your waist and thighs!" Wearing "weight-reducing" clothing or items such as these results in a temporary displacement of tissue or loss of water from the tissue, *not* a permanent loss of body fat. When you remove the item, the tissue soon regains its original shape; as soon as you drink, the water is replaced.

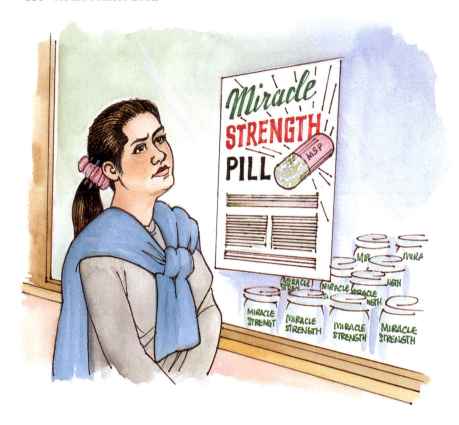

Choosing Exercise Equipment and Programs Wisely

A little background work and common sense on your part should allow you to select safe, effective equipment that meets both your fitness needs and your budget. Whenever possible, try out any equipment and preview any videos before you make a purchase.

Use the checklists that follow to help you decide which fitness equipment, center, book, or video is right for you. Compare several items. Don't buy equipment just because you've seen it advertised on TV or because the salesperson says it's "the best." Try it out to determine whether it feels right to you, whether you will use it, and whether you have room for it.

Choosing Equipment for Cardiorespiratory Endurance

Comfort and Effectiveness

- Is it easy to get onto and off of?
- Can it be adjusted to fit my body (seat height, frame length, foot rests, stride length, handlebars, etc.)?
- Are there controls that allow me to adjust the workload?
- Is it comfortable enough that I could use it for 30 minutes or more?

Reliability

- Can it support my weight?
- Is it sturdy, with a rigid frame that doesn't wobble when I use it?
- Are the gauges and controls easy to operate? What if they break?

Ease of Use and Maintenance

- Can I assemble it, or will the dealer do it for me?
- Can I change the resistance or any of the settings easily? Will they stay in the same place I put them?
- Where can I get the equipment repaired if it breaks?

Cost

- How much does it cost?
- Does the price include shipping or a warranty?
- Can I afford it?
- What are the alternatives if I don't buy it?

Choosing Home Weight-Training Equipment

Comfort and Effectiveness

- Does the equipment fit my body?
- Can I adjust the weights so I can work with them as I progress from a beginning to an experienced exerciser?
- Are the exercise positions comfortable?
- Is the equipment padded where I want it to be?
- Does the equipment work all my muscles?

Reliability

- Is the equipment sturdy (no wobbling or loose weights)?
- Do the weights move smoothly (no sticking or jerking)?
- Are additional weights or attachments available?

Ease of Use and Maintenance

- Is it easy to assemble?
- Do I have to buy any special attachments or make adjustments to my home?
- Is it easy to change the weights?
- If it breaks, where can I get the equipment serviced or maintained?

Cost

- What does it cost?
- Does the price include shipping or a warranty?
- Can I afford it?
- What are the alternatives if I do not buy the equipment?

Choosing a Fitness Center

Comfort and Convenience

- Is it close to my home or work?
- Are the hours convenient?
- Is daycare available if I need it?
- Would I be comfortable exercising with the other clients?
- Will I make time to get to the center?

Effectiveness

- Does it have all the equipment and services I want (treadmills, weights, pool, aerobic classes)?
- Is there enough equipment?
- Are locker facilities adequate?
- Is the staff friendly, knowledgeable, and available to assist me?
- Are the personnel certified? By whom?
- Are new members given an orientation including a fitness screening?

Maintenance

- Is the facility clean, secure, and ventilated?
- Is the equipment maintained?
- Are the safety and emergency procedures adequate?

Cost

- Is there a trial or an introductory period?
- Can I afford the membership?
- Can I get my money back if I discontinue my membership?
- What are the alternatives if I do not join?

Choosing a Fitness Book or Video

Comfort and Convenience

- Is it appropriate for my age, health status, and level of fitness?
- Does it provide safety guidelines, such as encouraging me to stop if something hurts?
- Can I use this workout regularly?
- Will I use this workout regularly?

Effectiveness

- Does the author or producer have appropriate fitness credentials or someone working with them who does?
- Does the book or video encourage improvement of all the fitness components?
- Does it include a warm-up and cool-down?
- Is it free from "miracle claims"?

Cost

- Can I afford the item?
- What is the alternative if I don't purchase this?

A Final Word

Increasing the amount of daily physical activity in your life is an important step in your commitment to leading a healthy lifestyle. Regular physical activity reduces your risk of many chronic diseases and improves your overall quality of life. We congratulate you on completing the ACSM Fitness Program and wish you good health as you continue a routine of daily physical activity.

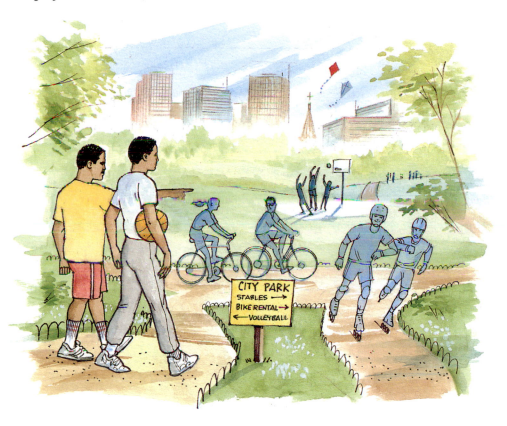

Index

About the Writing Team

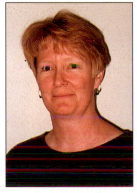

Susan M. Puhl, PhD, is experienced in designing, implementing, and evaluating fitness activities for individuals of all ages and abilities. Previously she worked in the exercise gerontology program at Penn State University, where she developed exercise programs for older adults and saw first-hand how appropriate physical activity can be used to prevent or decrease many age-related changes. Currently Susan is an associate professor of physical education and coordinator of adult fitness at the State University of New York (SUNY) College at Cortland. In addition to teaching and supervising students, Susan has developed a program of physical fitness testing and exercise programming for the faculty, staff, and students of SUNY at Cortland.

Susan is a member of the Certification and Education Committee of the American College of Sports Medicine (ACSM), and she is on the advisory board of the *ACSM's Health and Fitness Journal.*

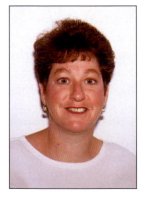

Madeline Paternostro-Bayles, PhD, has worked as a clinical exercise program director in a wide variety of settings during her career. She has served as co-director of Cardiac Rehabilitation at Allegheny General Hospital, administrative director of the Preventive Cardiology Program at the University of Pittsburgh Medical Center, and as director of the Cardiopulmonary

Rehabilitation Program at the University of Pittsburgh Medical Center. She is now an assistant professor in the department of physical education, health and sport at Indiana University of Pennsylvania.

Madeline received a PhD in exercise physiology from the University of Pittsburgh in 1985. In addition to being a fellow of the American College of Sports Medicine (ACSM), she is a past member of the ACSM's Certification and Education Committee and past president of the ACSM's Mid-Atlantic Chapter. She also is a fellow of the American Association of Cardiovascular and Pulmonary Rehabilitation.

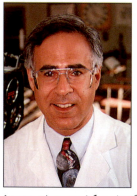

Barry Franklin, PhD, has served as the director of Cardiac Rehabilitation and Exercise Laboratories at William Beaumont Hospital in Royal Oak, Michigan since 1985. He is also a professor of physiology at Wayne State University School of Medicine in Detroit, Michigan. In addition to being a past vice president of the American College of Sports Medicine (ACSM), Barry is past president of the American Association of Cardiovascular and Pulmonary Rehabilitation and of the American Heart Association of Michigan. He is currently a member of the Governor's Council on Sports and Physical Fitness in Michigan.

Barry earned his PhD in physiology from Penn State University. A prolific writer, he has written more than 250 articles for professional and consumer publications and authored or coauthored six books on health and fitness. Three of his reports have been published in the prestigious *Journal of the American Medical Association.* Franklin served as editor-in-chief of the *Journal of Cardiopulmonary Rehabilitation* from 1990 to 1995. Currently he is an associate editor and columnist for the *ACSM's Health and Fitness Journal,* and he serves on the editorial/review boards of the *American Journal of Health Promotion, American Journal of Cardiology,* and *Physician and Sportsmedicine.*

Effective Training Options
from Beginning to Advanced

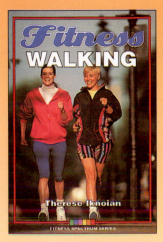

Fitness Walking
Therese Iknoian

1995 • Paper • 168 pp • Item PIKN0553
ISBN 0-87322-553-8 • $15.95 ($21.95 Canadian)

Create a walking program tailored to your needs and abilities.

Fitness Weight Training
Thomas R. Baechle, EdD, CSCS, and Roger Earle, MA, CSCS

1995 • Paper • 176 pp • Item PBAE0445
ISBN 0-87322-445-0 • $15.95 ($21.95 Canadian)

Design a custom-made weight training program that fits your goals.

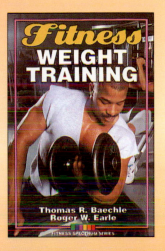

FITNESS SPECTRUM SERIES

A practical and flexible approach to training. Each book is packed with workouts, color-coded by level of difficulty, that you can use to set up a personalized training program or to add variety to your exercise routine.

Also available in the Fitness Spectrum Series:

Fitness Aerobics
Fitness Aquatics
Fitness Cross-Training
Fitness Cycling
Fitness In-Line Skating
Fitness Running
Fitness Stepping

Human Kinetics
The Premier Publisher for Sports & Fitness
http://www.humankinetics.com/

Prices subject to change.

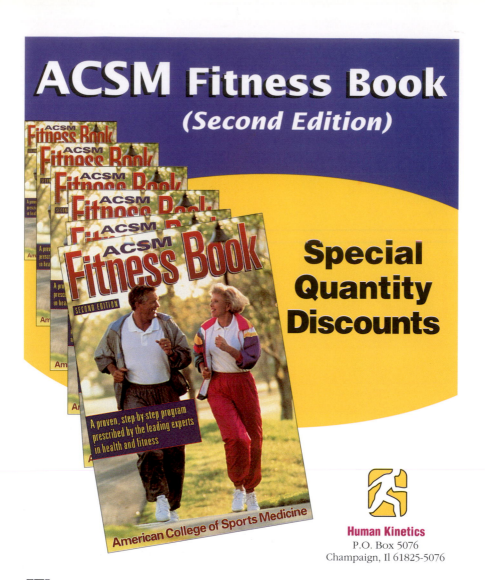

ACSM Fitness Book
(Second Edition)

American College of Sports Medicine

A proven, step-by-step program prescribed by the leading experts in health and fitness

Special Quantity Discounts

Human Kinetics
P.O. Box 5076
Champaign, Il 61825-5076

Would you like to make copies of this practical and informative book available to your employees, colleagues, or clients? Human Kinetics offers a special discount program that makes the second edition of the *ACSM Fitness Book* an affordable option for you.

Discounts start when you order a minimum of 10 books. Purchase larger quantities and receive more substantial savings! Call us using the appropriate telephone number below and ask about our special quantity discounts for the *ACSM Fitness Book* (Second Edition).